The Abdominal Exercise Bible: Ab Exercises For Core Strength And A Flat Belly

By Anthony Anholt

Discover other fitness titles by Anthony Anholt on Kindle:

The Isometric Exercise Bible
The Bodyweight Exercise Bible

Disclaimer

The exercises and advice contained within this course may be too strenuous or dangerous for some people and the reader(s) should consult a physician before engaging in them. The author and publisher of this book are not responsible in any manner whatsoever for any injury which may occur through reading and following the instructions herein.

Table Of Contents

Abdominal Exercises And You	3
6-Pack Abs Vs Conditioned Muscles	5
Core Training Explained	7
Mandatory Core Training Exercises	11
Abdominal Exercises For The Front	19
Core Training For The Side	59
Core Exercises For The Back	87
FAQ	124
Further Reading	129
About The Author/Models	130
One Last Thing	131

Abdominal Exercises And You

The secret of getting ahead is getting started. -Mark Twain

To most people few things scream health and fitness more than a tight and toned mid-section. A flat belly, regardless of whether you actually have a 6-pack, is youthful, sexy and desirable. This is why so many of us engage in ab exercises of various kinds and is probably the reason you are reading this book right now. Am I right?

However the benefits of having real core strength go far beyond mere appearance. The muscles in and around your stomach, otherwise known as your core, support your entire body. The health advantages you will enjoy if you keep this section of your body strong and healthy are many. Here are just a few of them:

* A program of abdominal exercises will help improve your digestion and elimination of food wastes. This is known as peristalsis, which is the process by which your systems move food through your body.

* Core exercises will help you improve your athletic performance in whatever sport you play. Your power, whether you're swinging a golf club or a tennis racquet, is centered in your abdominals.

* Core training will help you greatly reduce or even eliminate lower back pain.

* Strong abdominal muscles will help improve your posture. Too many of us have poor posture as we sit at desk jobs all day.

* Performing stomach exercises, particularly the simple breathing exercises you are about to learn, will improve your energy levels. In many Eastern disciplines like yoga and the martial arts the core is considered to be an energy center. The more core exercises you do the more you will agree with the wisdom of this view.

* Having strong abdominals will actually reduce the pressure on your joints. Weak stomach muscles often force other muscles and joints to compensate in order to stabilize your body. Strengthening your abdominals with core exercises will help to alleviate this issue.

* Exercise in general, which obviously includes core exercises, can help to reduce common conditions like cholesterol and blood sugar. It can even slow down or outright prevent arthritis and can even help with mild depression.

* By increasing your muscle mass abdominal exercises can even help you with fat burning and weight loss.

6-Pack Abs Vs Conditioned Muscles

Your waistline is your lifeline – Paul Bragg

Despite all I have just said about the many health benefits that derive from having a trained core, I know that many of you will still cite "getting a 6-pack" as your primary reason for performing these abdominal exercises. There is nothing wrong with this, but you should just know that this is not the primary purpose of this book. What concerns me the most, as an author and exercise enthusiast, is to possess conditioned muscles, particularly in the core area. To me conditioned muscle is synonymous with highly functional muscle that allows you to move your body in all angles and directions. Conditioned muscles give you energy and pep, strength and endurance, not just looks.

Here's the truth. Super ripped abdominals are usually the result of some combination of genetics and super strict dieting. I've seen drug addicts with abs that are completely ripped. Are they healthy? I don't think so. Does this mean that you cannot achieve the vaunted 6-pack? Not in the least. It just means that you will (unless you are genetically blessed) have to follow a fairly strict diet along with the stomach exercises you are about to learn. There is an old fitness aphorism that goes something like this: "You get stronger in the gym, but you get leaner in the kitchen." This means cutting way back on the sugar and junk food and starting to eat a healthy diet. There is no way around it.

If you don't want to watch your diet religiously should you not even bother with these core training exercises? Of course you should. You don't need five percent body fat to look fantastic or be fit. By strengthening your core muscles you will look younger and feel better no matter what. I suggest you always aim for conditioned muscle over looks. It's a worthwhile goal.

Core Training Explained

Don't stop trying just because you've hit a wall.
Progress is progress no matter how small -
Unknown

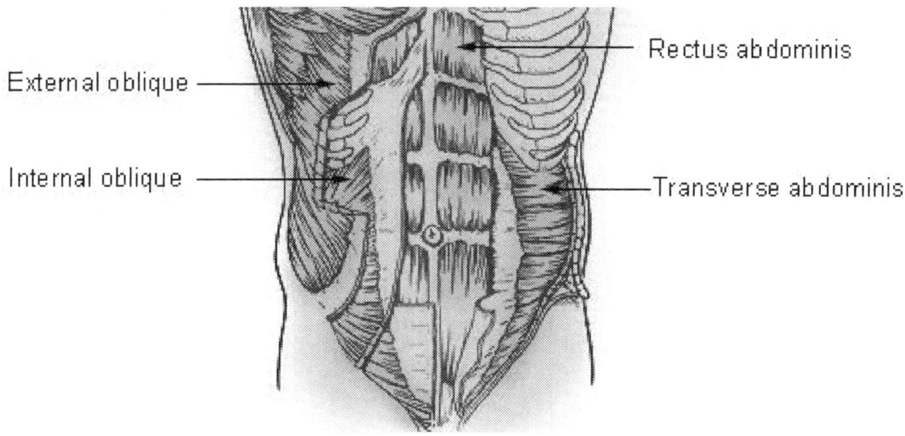

The following are the abdominal muscle groups that make up what people commonly call "The Core":

Rectus Abdominis – This is the outermost layer of muscle on your abdomen. These are the muscles you see when you have a 6-pack.

Transverse Abdominis – These muscles are typically used to pull your body down. If you place your hands on your sides and cough, you can feel these muscles.

External Oblique – This is the primary muscle you use when you twist, bend, or rotate your body from the torso.

Internal Oblique – This muscle exists below the external oblique where it assists the external oblique in moving the torso. It also helps with the process of breathing.

The Abdominal Exercises Bible core-training program is divided into sections in order to ensure that all of these muscles are given a thorough workout. The first section is made up of three exercises that should be done with every abdominal workout. Two of the exercises are actually deep breathing exercises that will energize you while simultaneously working your internal oblique and transverse abdominis muscle. These exercises by themselves will go a long way to helping you accomplish your goal of having a flat belly. The reason for this is that most stomach exercises rarely work these muscles. However when they are strong and developed they will tighten your entire mid-section. The other sections are divided into core strength exercises for the front, back and side of your midsection. What you will do here is pick one or two exercises and perform them. Here's what a typical workout might look like:

Mandatory Core Training Exercises

Tai Chi Waist Turner

Isometric Stomach Flattener

The Vacuum

Abdominal Exercises For The Front

Leg Circles

Tuck Ups

Abdominal Exercises For the Side

Oblique Curls

Advanced Beach Scissors

Abdominal Exercises For The Back

Reverse Leg Lifts

Torso Lifts

Again, this is only a sample. Every core training session you do should contain the three ab exercises mentioned (Tai Chi Waist Turner, Isometric Stomach Flattener and The Vacuum). With the others you can pick which ones you want to do. The exercises in these sections are arranged roughly from easiest to hardest so, if you are a beginner, start at the beginning. If you are more advanced go to the back of the section to find more challenging exercises. How often should you do this program? You can perform it everyday if you wish although this isn't necessary. If you perform these core exercises three to four times a week while watching your diet you'll possess a flat belly in no time.

With that the groundwork has been laid and we're ready to begin. Let's get started.

Mandatory Core Training Exercises

Energy and persistence conquer all things. - Benjamin Franklin

This section is made up of the three ab exercises you should perform every time you engage in core training. The Tai Chi waist turner is a great exercise for energizing and warming up your body. The isometric stomach flattener and vacuum are great stomach exercises that utilize your breath in order to work the internal abdominal muscles that often get ignored.

Tai Chi Waist Turner

This exercise is excellent for warming up your core. In addition, it will increase the flexibility in your waist, massage your internal organs and help to give you a flat belly. It is an extremely simply yet effective exercise.

1. Begin with your feet shoulder width apart and your arms hanging loosely by your sides.
2. Keep your feet planted as you begin to twist your entire spine from side to side. As you do so, allow the centrifugal force you are generating to move your arms freely.
3. Each time you have twisted as far as you comfortably can to one side, allow your hands to gently slap you in the kidneys. This will give them a gentle massage.
4. Perform 50 – 100 repetitions.

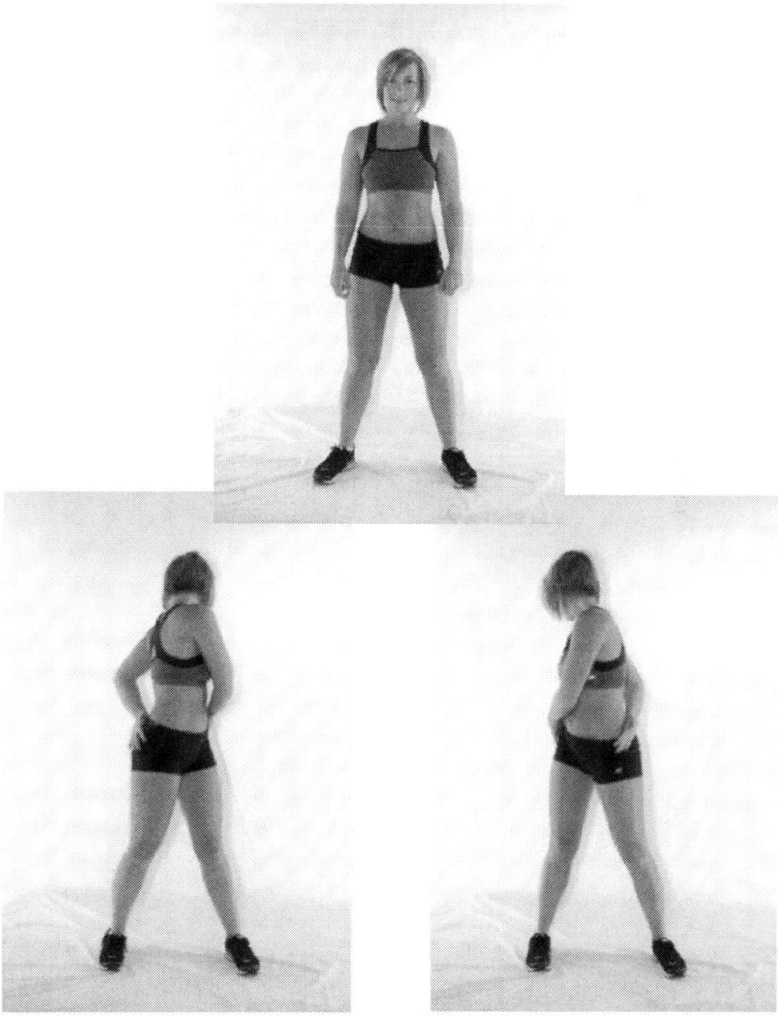

Isometric Stomach Flattener

The Isometric Stomach Flattener may well be the best exercise you can do in order to gain a flat belly and real core strength yet it is seldom taught. The reason it is so effective is it works two muscle groups that most abdominal exercises barely touch, namely the transversus abdominus and internal oblique muscles. The great advantage of working these muscles is that they are the ones that, when trained, effortlessly keep your gut sucked in. This abdominal exercise can also be done seated at your desk, on the bus or while you are standing at a stoplight. If you take on this attitude of performing this abs exercise anywhere you have a few seconds, you'll have a tighter and more functional midsection in no time.

1. Inhale through your nose for three seconds in order to completely fill your lungs. As you do so, keep your stomach muscles gently flexed but do not overly exert yourself.
2. Clench your fists as you breathe out hard through your mouth for 7 seconds. As you do so, place your tongue on the roof of your mouth so that you make a soft "SSSSSS" sound almost like a snake. As you exhale in this manner you should be flexing your stomach muscles as hard as you can.
3. As you are performing this exercise actively picture in your mind how your stomach muscles are flexing and working.
4. Repeat this action by again breathing in through your nose while slightly relaxing your stomach muscles.

At no time during this exercise should you ever hold your breath. When you start performing this exercise you may feel somewhat lightheaded. If so take a break until the feeling passes.

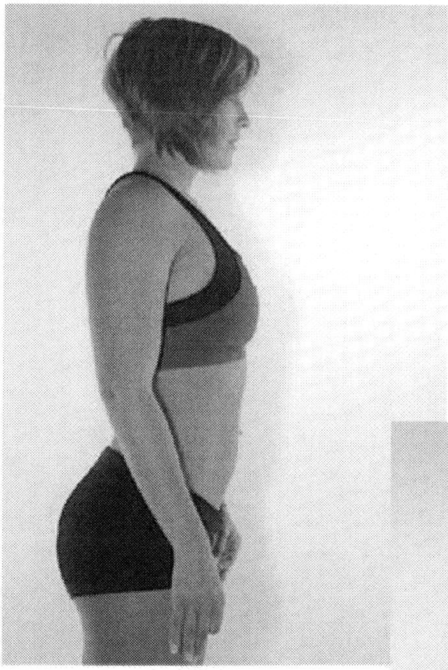

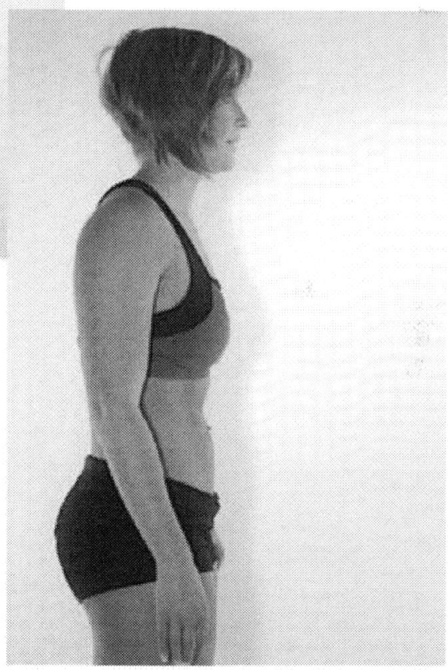

The Vacuum

This ab exercise, along with the isometric stomach flattener, will reduce your waistline and improve the functioning of your digestive system. This is one of the few exercises where it is necessary to hold your breath. Remember though that if you feel faint at anytime, take a break and breathe normally until the feeling passes.

1. Begin by bending over with your hands resting on your knees.
2. Slowly exhale all the air from your lungs through your mouth.
3. Once your lungs are empty, rise slightly and lift your diaphragm while pulling your stomach in.
4. Hold for a count of 6 seconds or longer.
5. Inhale through your nose and catch your breath.
6. Repeat this exercise 5 to 10 times.

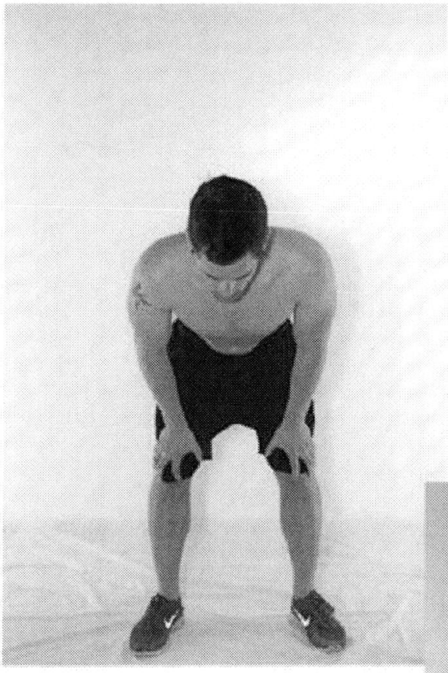

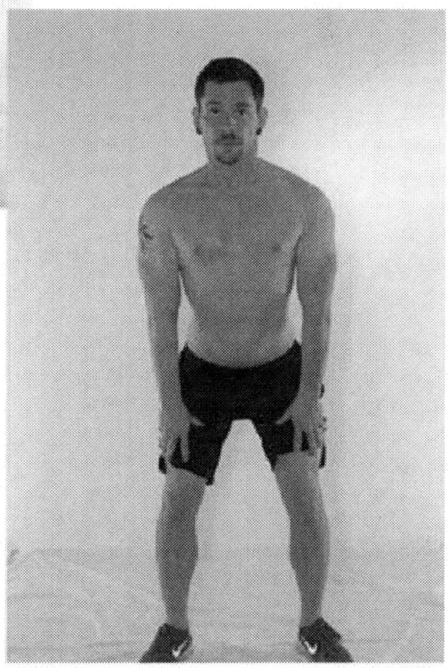

Abdominal Exercises For The Front

You don't have to go fast ... you just have to go
- Unknown

Although these stomach exercises focus on the front of your abdominal muscles you will likely feel secondary effects elsewhere. The reason for this is all of these core training exercises treat your abdomen as a unit. The result is that if one muscle group is relatively weak compared to another group it is the weaker group that will get most of the work. This is the key to getting a functional midsection that will keep you strong and healthy for life. Your task now is to pick one or two of the ab exercises that follow and perform them. The easier exercises are at the beginning and they then progress in difficulty from there.

The Gut Sucker

The gut sucker is a beginner's exercise yet it much harder than it looks. The main reason is that it is one of the few exercises you perform without breathing. As this is the case, you may find it quite difficult at first. If at anytime feel out of breath or lightheaded stop immediately. At first you may only be able to do 3 to 5. Keep at it until you can perform 15 or more on a single breath.

1. Begin with your legs a little wider than hip width apart and your knees slightly bent. Bend over at your waist and place your hands on your thighs for support.
2. Exhale all of the air from your lungs through your mouth. As you do so, suck your belly button in toward your spine.
3. While holding your breath pump your belly button in and out as many times as you can.
4. You may repeat this exercise 2 or 3 times, if you wish.

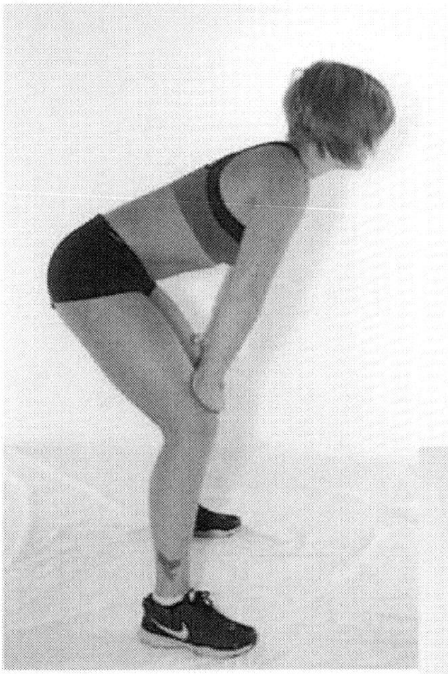

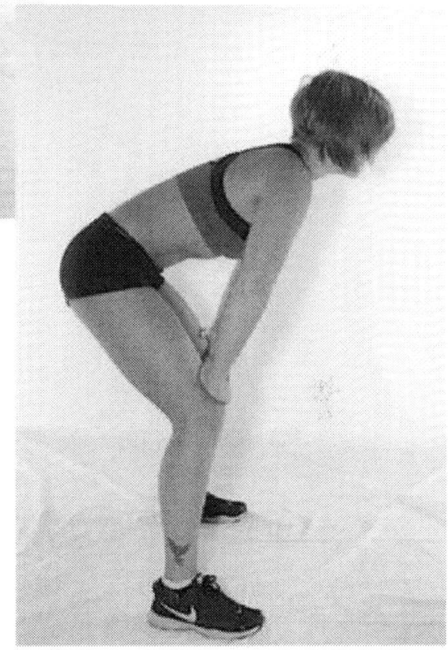

Standing Knee Raises

The balancing this exercise requires will not only build real core strength but will develop your leg muscles as well.

1. Begin by standing with your feet roughly shoulder width apart.

2. Raise both of your arms parallel to the floor for balance.

3. Inhale through your nose as you raise your left knee as high as possible.

   Hold it in this position for a count of three.

4. Exhale through your mouth as you lower your left leg to the ground.

5. Repeat this motion with your right leg.

6. Continue alternating legs until fatigued.

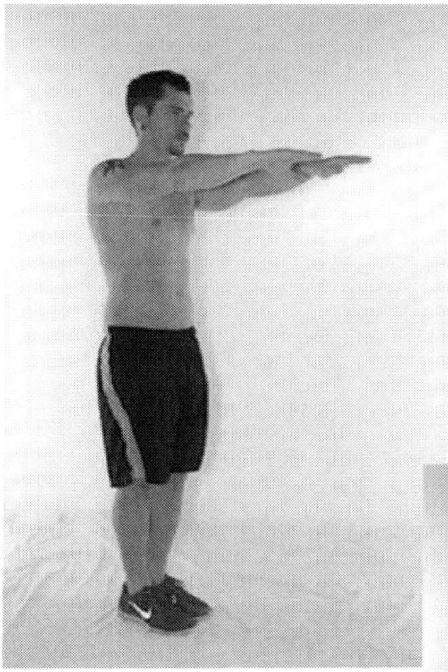

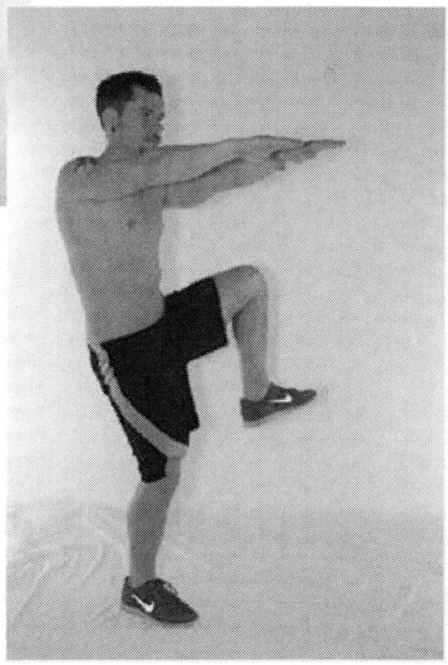

The Woodchopper

Due to the motion involved some people may find this ab exercise hard on their lower backs. When performing it, make sure you keep your abs tight at all times to support your lower back. If back issues persist, I suggest you skip this exercise all together.

1. Begin in a wide stance with your fingers interlaced above your head.
2. Exhale through your mouth as you bring your hands between your legs as if you are chopping wood. Remember to keep your back straight and your abs tight as you do this.
3. Inhale through your nose as you raise your body back to the starting position.
4. Repeat this motion 6 to 10 times.

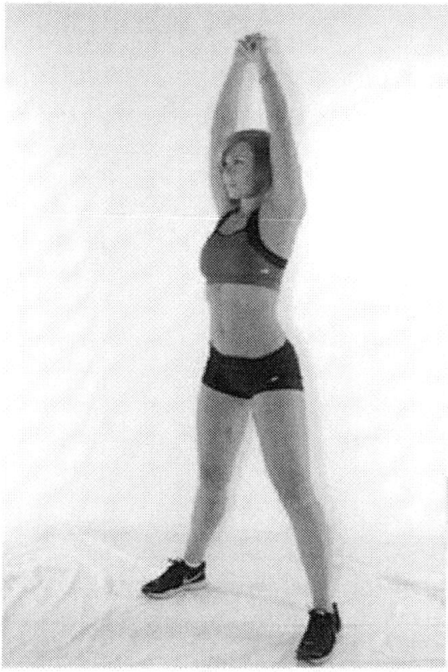

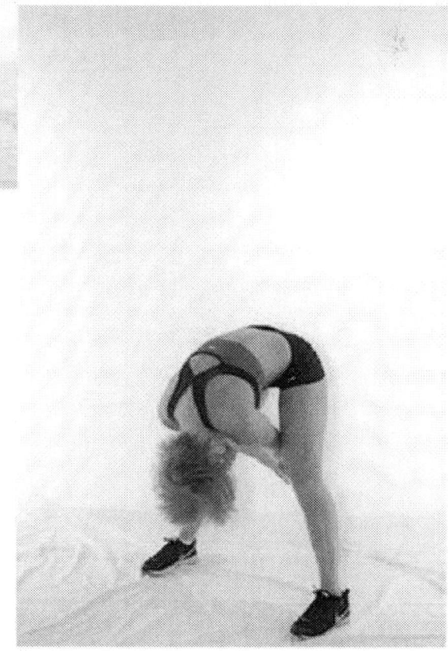

Standing Bicycle

Most people find this exercise to be easier than bicycles performed on the ground. However it has the added benefit of improving you balance at the same time.

1. Begin with your feet shoulder width apart and your fingers interlaced behind your head. This is the starting position.
2. Exhale through your mouth as you raise your left knee to your stomach while bringing your right elbow to the outside of your left knee.
3. Return to the starting position while breathing in through your nose.
4. Repeat this motion using your right knee and left elbow.

Try to do this 3 -5 more times. When you work up to 10 you are doing well.

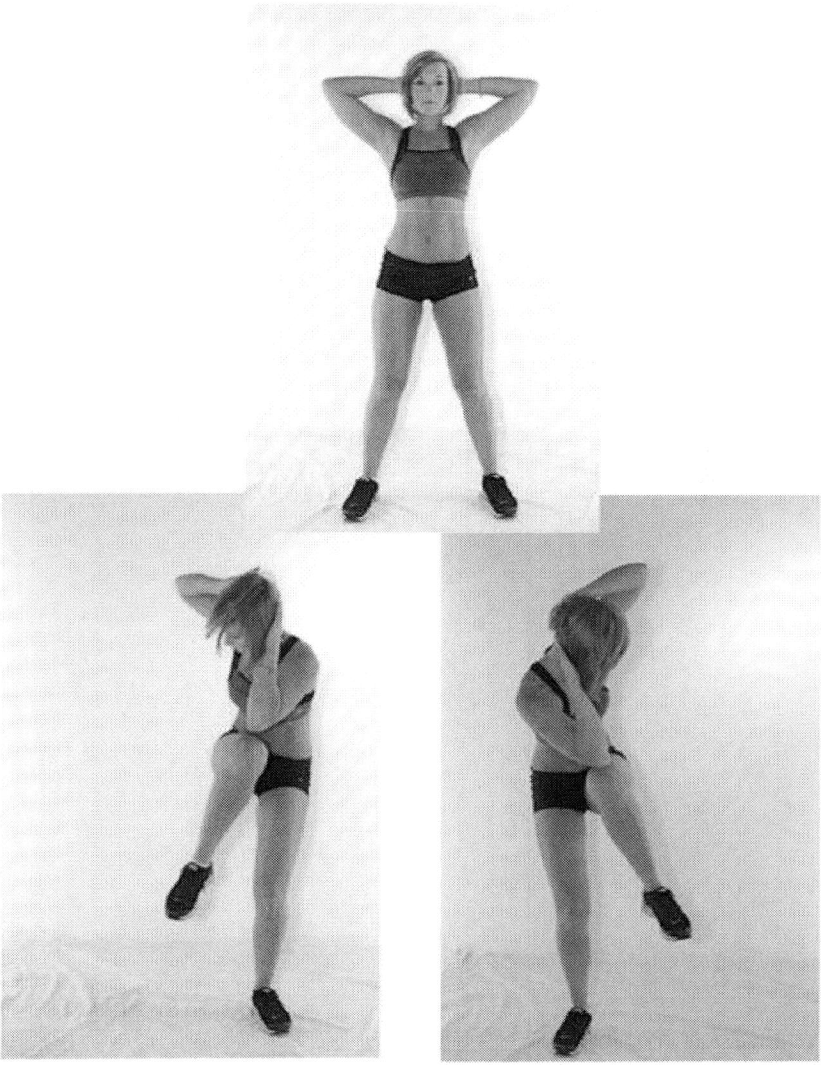

Easy Boat

This is a gentle core exercise that will also help you with your sense of balance.

1. Begin by sitting on the floor with your knees bent in front of you. Your feet should be on the floor.
2. Place your hands on the back of your thighs.
3. While maintaining your balance, raise your shins off the ground so that they are parallel to the floor while arching your spine.
4. Breathe in through your nose and exhale through your mouth.
5. Hold this position for a slow count of 5 to 10.

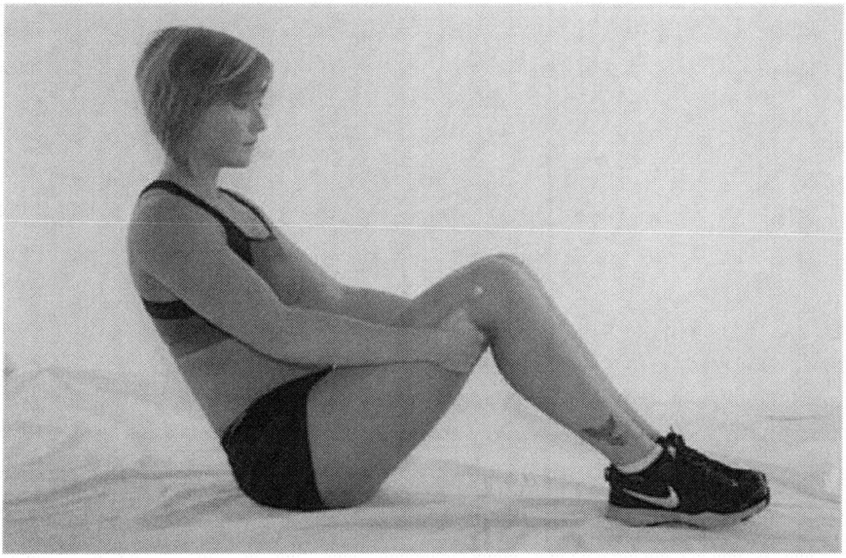

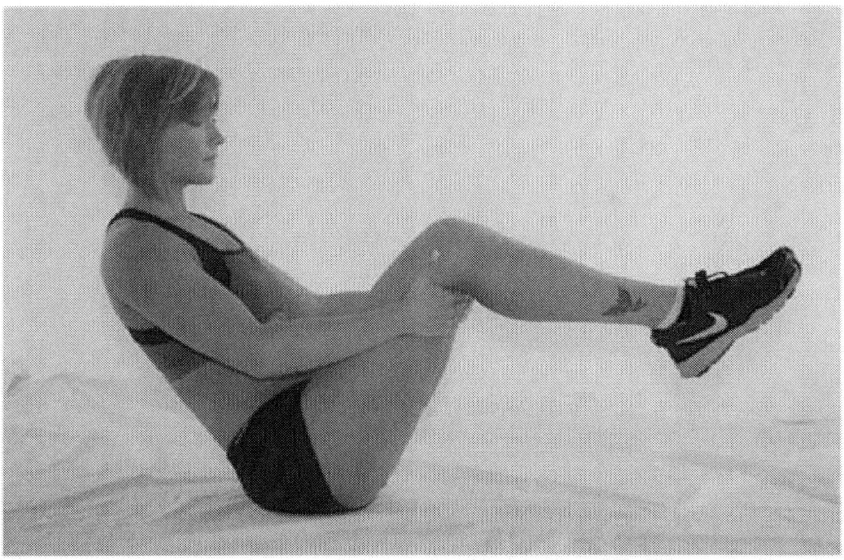

One Legged Boat

This ab exercise is an intermediate step on your way to performing a full boat.

1. Begin with your knees bent and your feet on the floor.
2. Place your hand on the back of your thighs.
3. While maintaining your balance, extend your right leg while keeping your left foot on the ground.
4. Arch your back and extend your arms.
5. Keep your stomach tight as you inhale through your nose and exhale through your mouth.
6. Hold this position for a count of 5 and then switch legs.

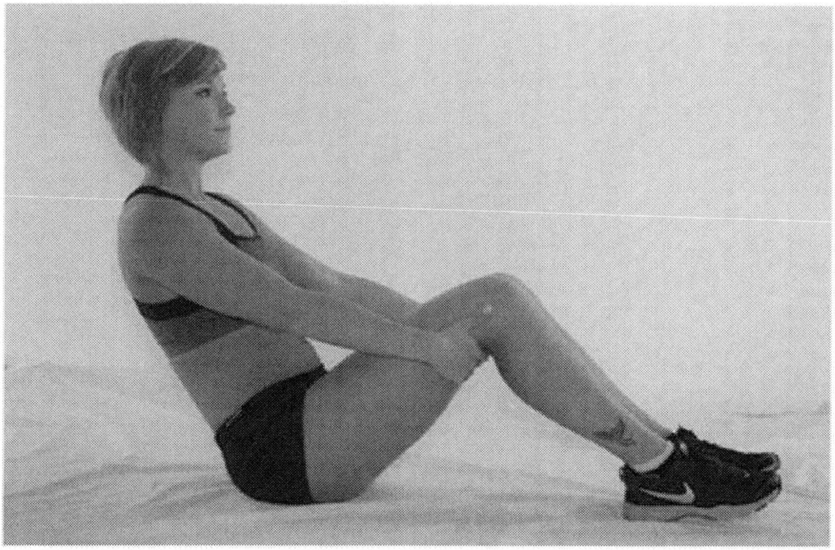

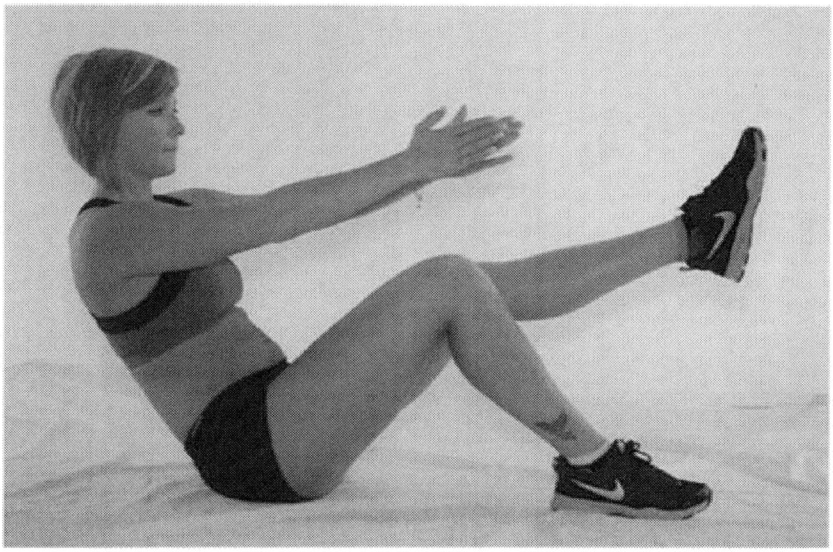

Full Boat

With this abdominal exercise you will be forced to use your core to maintain your balance. This forces your abdominal muscles to work in ways that using a machine of some kind simply does not.

1. Begin with your knees bent and your feet on the floor.
2. Place your hands on the back of your thighs.
3. Arch your back and suck in your stomach muscles while you raise both legs off the floor. Your torso and legs should form a roughly 45-degree angle.
4. Extend your arms so they are parallel to the ground.
5. Inhale through your nose and exhale through your mouth as you hold this position for a slow count of 5 – 10.

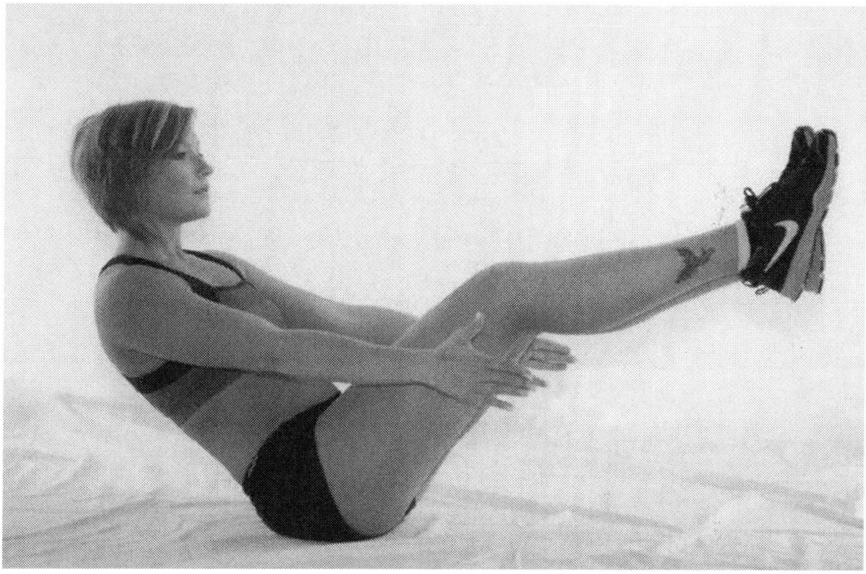

String Pull

With this ab exercise you will be working your core by pretending that you are a marionette. It is a simple idea yet very effective in crafting a flat belly.

1. Begin by lying on your back with your knees bent and feet on the floor. Your arms should be straight beside you with your palms on the ground.
2. As you exhale through your mouth, press your belly button to the floor while slightly lifting your torso and bringing your chin to your chest. With this movement you are trying to press your lower spine to the floor as best you can.
3. Inhale through your nose as you raise your right hand toward your head. As you do so you will simultaneously bring your right knee to your chest. To help you do this, imagine that your knee is attached to your hand with a string.
4. Lower your right knee and hand back to the ground.
5. Repeat this motion with your left leg and hand.
6. Repeat this cycle until fatigued.

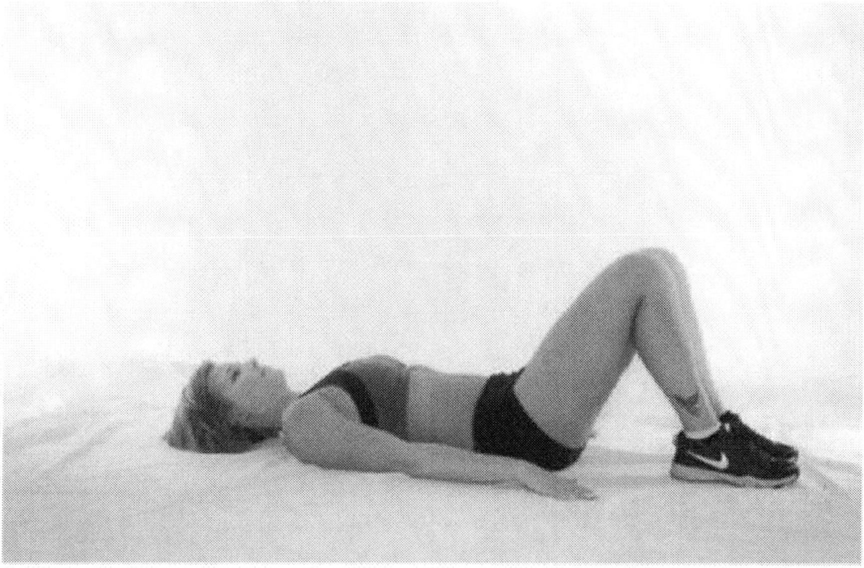

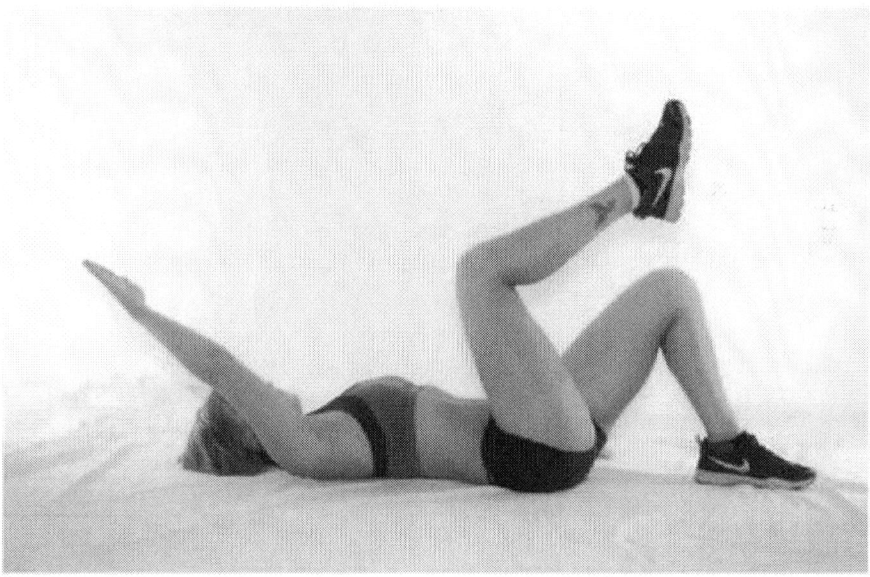

Leg Circles

With this core exercise you will be tracing circles in the air with your feet.

1. Begin by lying flat on your back with your legs straight in the air.
2. Separate your legs so that they are approximately 12 inches apart.
3. Move your legs so that each foot makes three small circles in the air.
4. Separate your legs a little more and then again trace three small circles in the air with your feet. The circles will be bigger this time than they were in the first set.
5. Separate your legs even more and make three even wider circles again.
6. Reverse direction and bring your legs in a little so that the three circles you make are smaller than the previous ones.
7. Finish by making the same small circles that you started with.

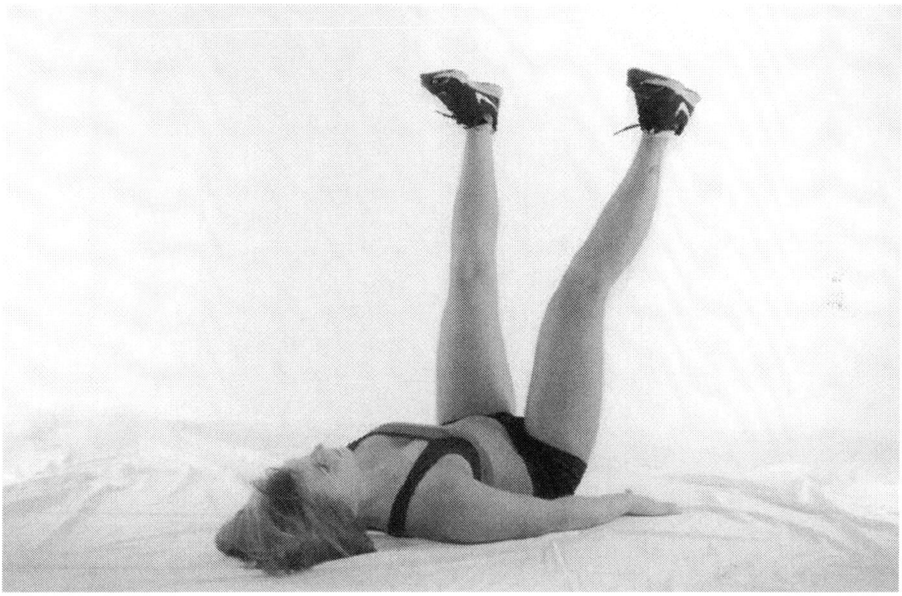

Yoga Sit-Ups

The classic sit-up that so many of us knew from high school isn't that effective simply because it is so easy to cheat by using your arms. This exercise looks easier but is actually more effective and is easier on your back, too.

1. Begin by lying on your back with your knees bent and your feet on the floor.
2. Place the palms of your hands on your legs straight in front of you and bring your chin toward your chest.
3. Exhale through your mouth as you press your belly to the floor while you simultaneously bring your hands toward your knees. This will lift your torso off the ground.
4. Hold this position for 3 seconds before lowering your torso back to the floor. Inhale through your nose as you do so.
5. Repeat 3 to 5 times or until fatigued.

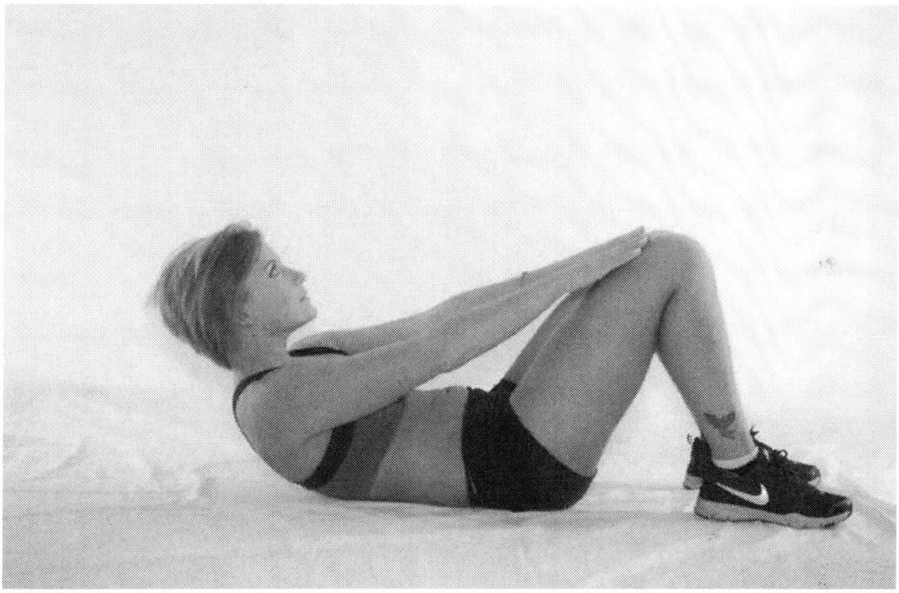

Tuck Ups

Tuck ups are a great abdominal exercise that will build great core strength and lean abs. They will also help you eliminate pain and weakness in your lower back.

1. Begin by lying on your back with your arms stretched out straight behind your head.
2. Take a deep breath through your nose as you tighten your abs and glutes.
3. Exhale through your mouth as you raise your upper body and legs simultaneously and bring them together into a tight tuck. The closer you get your legs to your torso the harder your abdominals are working.
4. Lower your legs and torso back to the ground as you breathe in through your nose.
5. Try to work up to doing 20 repetitions in a row.

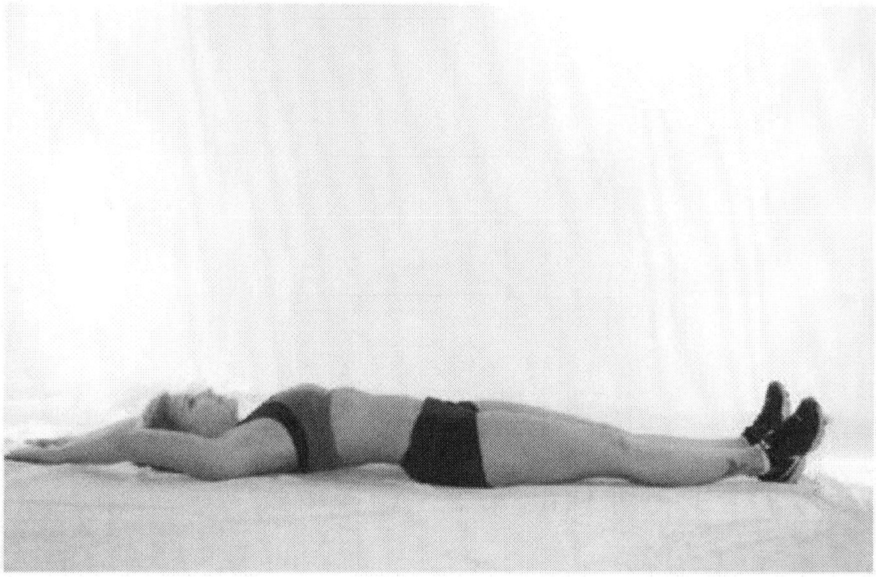

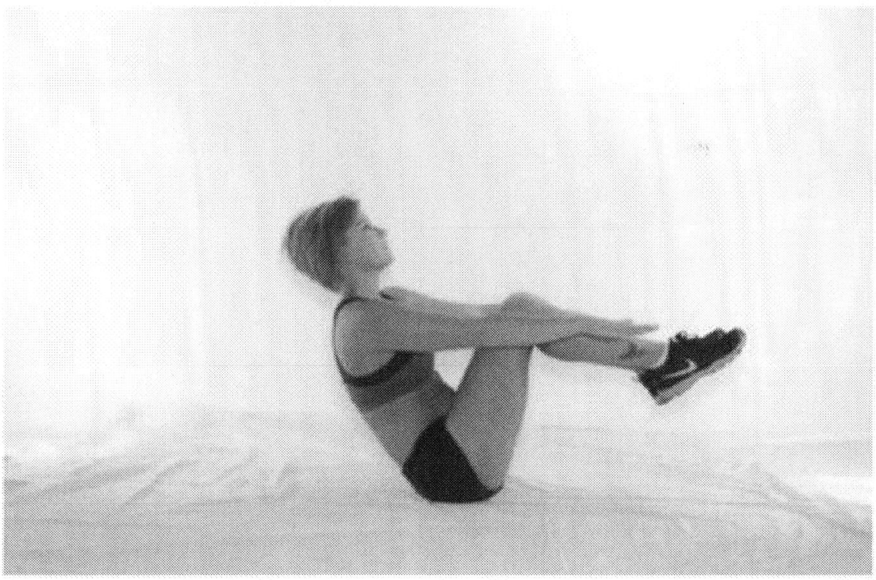

Hollow Ups

This ab exercise will develop the whole body, as well as, build tremendous core strength along with your abdominal wall. As a bonus it will also shape and tone your legs, as well.

1. Begin with your back on the floor, legs together and your arms straight overhead.
2. Exhale through your mouth as you raise your arms and legs simultaneously into a hollow position. Your goal is to shape your body like a rocker on the bottom of a rocking chair.
3. Lower your arms and legs back to the starting position as you breathe in through your nose.
4. Repeat this movement 15 times or until fatigued.

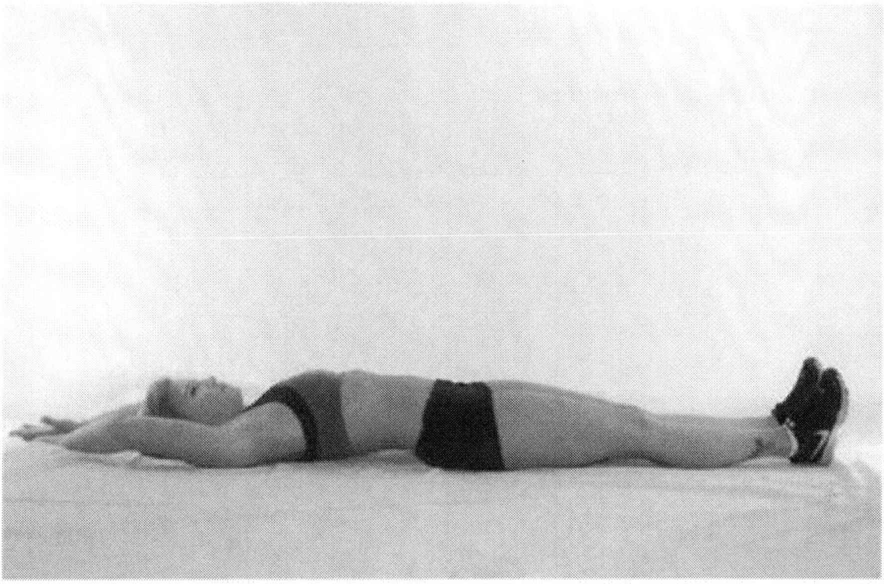

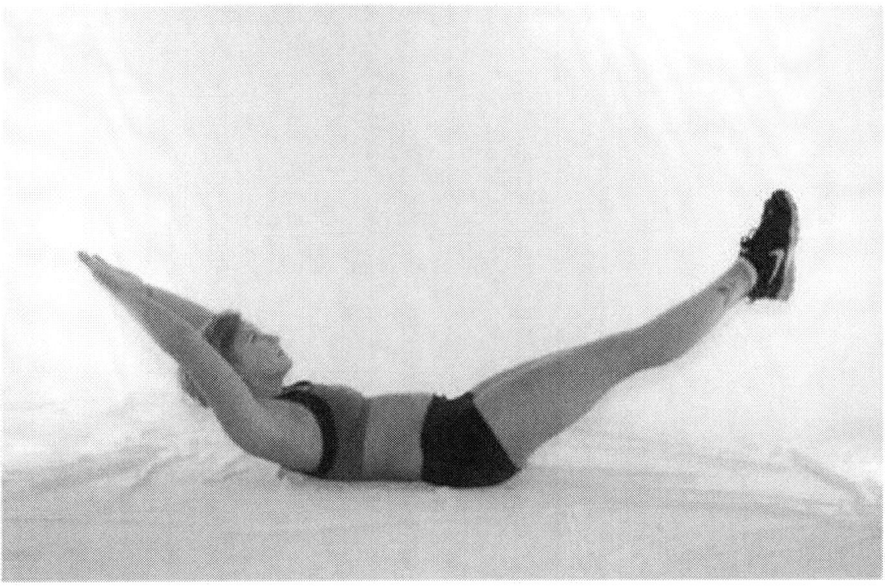

Hollow Body Rocks

This core exercise will go a long way in giving you a flat belly and a long sinewy body. When you do them correctly by focusing on every muscle, don't be surprised if you are huffing and puffing too.

1. Begin with your back on the floor, legs together and your arms straight overhead.
2. Exhale through your mouth as you raise your arms and legs simultaneously into a hollow position. Your goal is to shape your body like a rocker on the bottom of a rocking chair.
3. Flex the muscles in your abs, butt and legs as you start to rock back and forth as if you were a rocker on the bottom of a rocking chair.
4. Breathe in through your nose and out through your mouth. Never hold your breath.
5. Try for 12 repetitions or until fatigued.

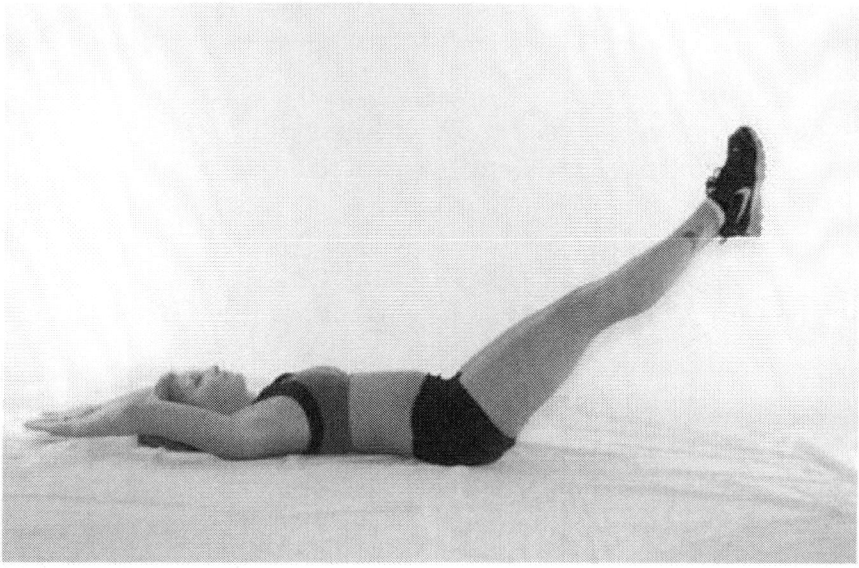

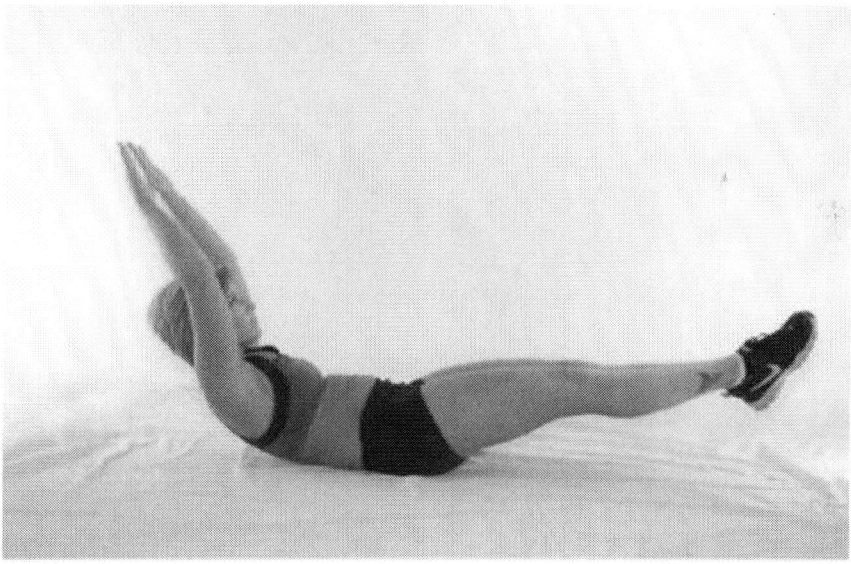

Leg Lifts

Performed correctly, leg lifts will strengthen and tone your lower abs. When performing this core exercise, always focus on feeling your abs working as opposed to using your hips. A variation is to perform this exercise with your head raised off the ground as this will help strengthen your neck.

1. Begin by lying on your back with your hands under your butt.
2. Raise your legs off the ground until they are at a 45 to 90 degree angle.
3. During the entire movement try to flex your legs straight while keeping your toes pointed. Try to keep your knees straight. Doing this will lengthen and tone your leg muscles.
4. Hold the "Up" position for 2 seconds before lowering your legs to just above the floor in a controlled manner.
5. Do until fatigued. When you can do 20 repetitions in a row, you are doing well.

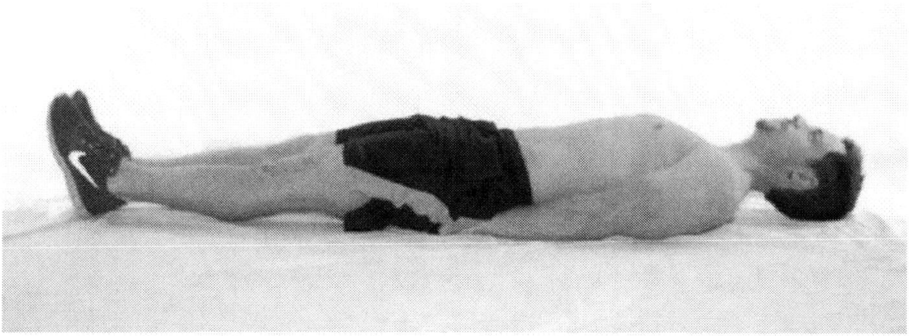

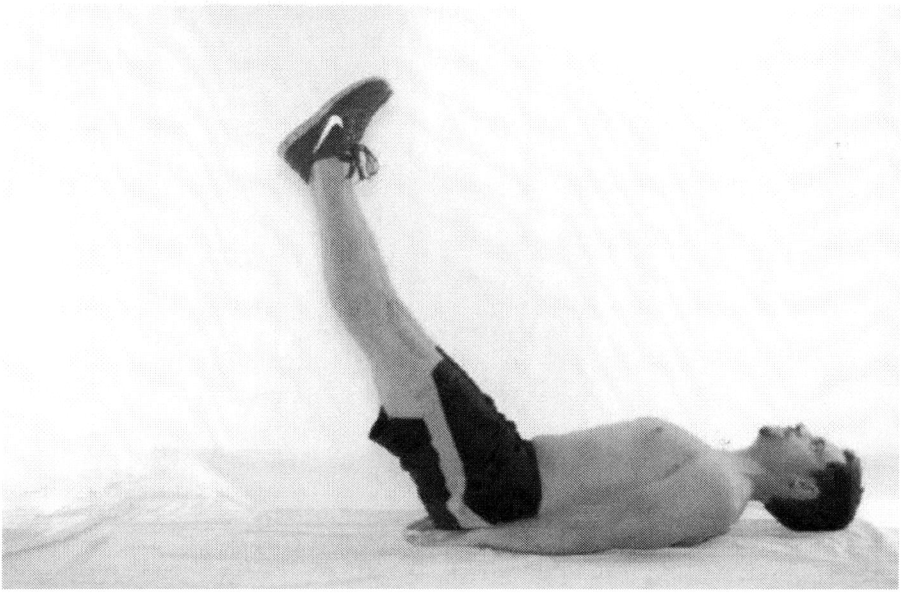

No Momentum Sit-Ups

This stomach exercise is performed slowly and deliberately, which makes it almost impossible to cheat. Your goal is to imitate a zombie or a vampire rising from the grave. It is this slow motion that will really strengthen your abdominals while giving you a flat belly.

1. Begin by lying on the floor with your arms by your sides.
2. Slowly start to raise your upper body off the ground using your abdominal muscles only. Your heels and legs should never come off the floor.
3. Continue to rise until your upper body is perpendicular to the floor.
4. Reverse direction and lower your upper body to the ground. Make sure you go slowly here as well - as you want to work your muscles in both directions.
5. Perform as many as you can until fatigued.

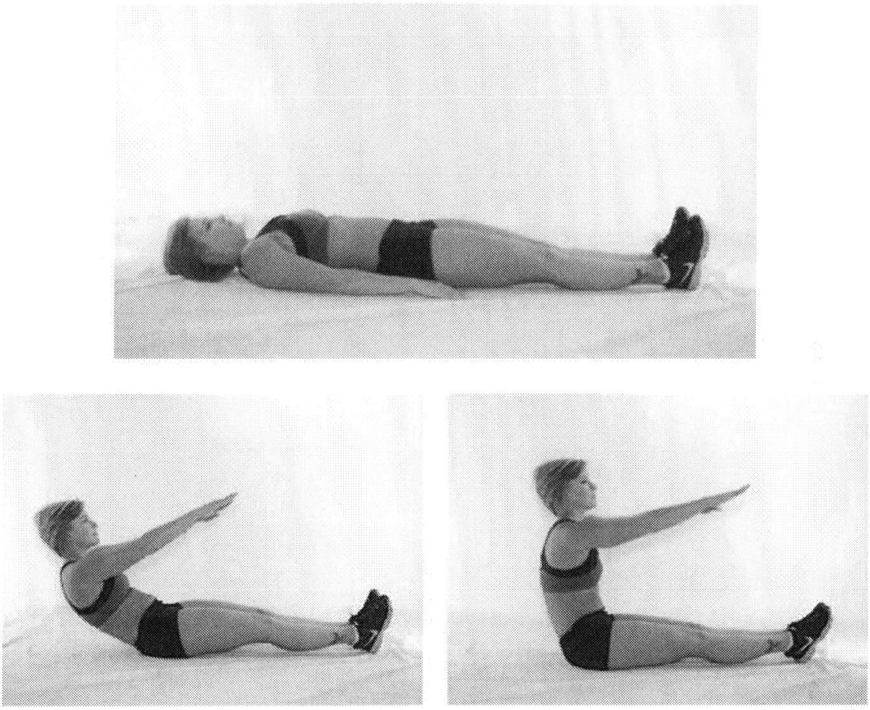

Toes Behind Head Leg Lifts

This is a great exercise for your abdominals that will also increase the flexibility of your back and legs. It will also help increase your circulation, massage your internal organs and aid in the digestive process.

1. Begin by lying flat on your back with your hands by your side and your legs straight.
2. Keeping your legs straight at all times point your toes and lift them all the way over your head.
3. Touch your toes to the ground behind you.
4. Return your legs back to the starting position.
5. Do as many repetitions as you can until fatigued.

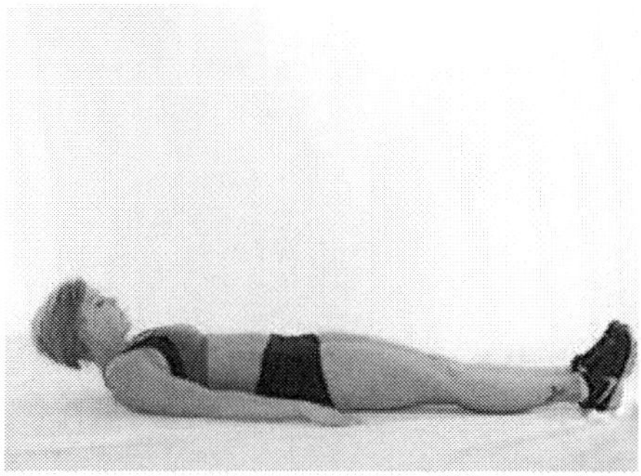

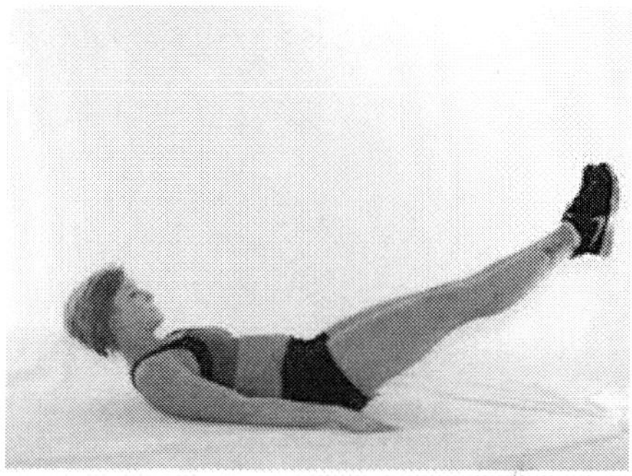

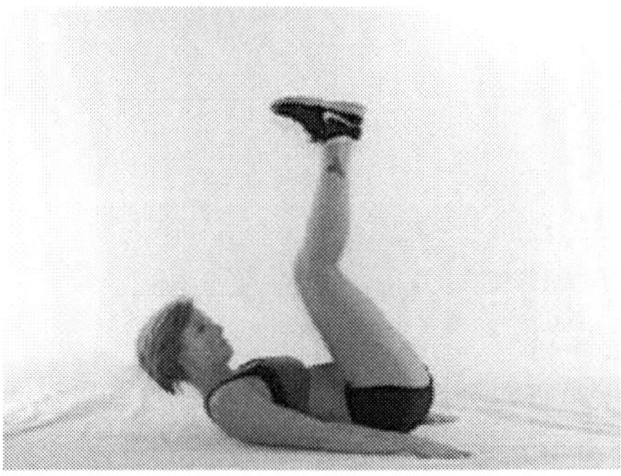

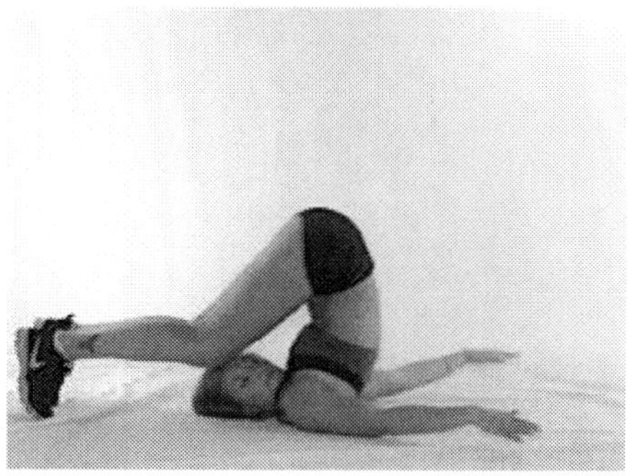

Leg Scissors

Leg scissors are a great core strength exercise that will not only work your abdominals, but will hit your inner and outer thighs, as well as, your hip flexors.

1. Begin by lying flat on your back with your legs straight and your arms by your side.
2. Tuck your chin into your chest as you simultaneously lift both legs about 6 inches off the floor. Your legs can either be straight or slightly bent.
3. Inhale through your nose as you open your legs wide.
4. Exhale through your mouth as you reverse direction and cross your legs.
5. Continue until fatigued. When you can do between 25 and 50 repetitions, you are doing well.
6. Remember to alternate the leg that goes under and over on each repetition.

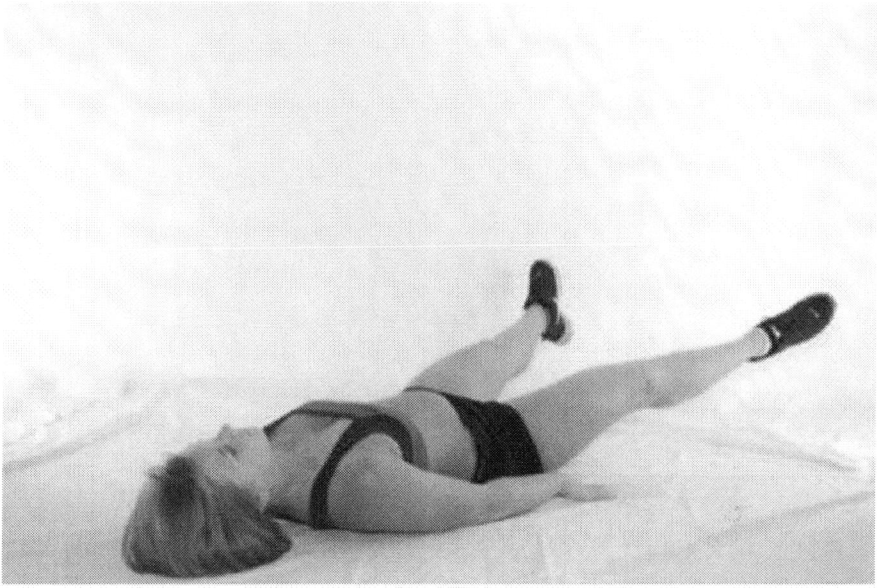

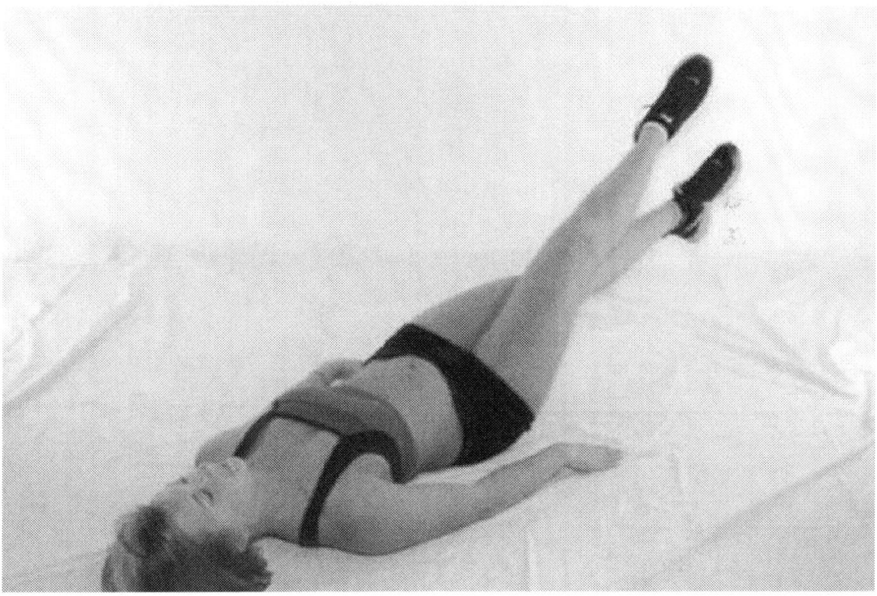

Butt Risers

This abdominal exercise will work your entire core with a focus on your lower abdomen. The act of lifting your body off the ground forces your large abdominal muscles to work, as well as, many smaller muscles in order for you to maintain your balance. If you wish to make this exercise easier, try bending your knees. To make it harder, keep your legs straight in the air.

1. Begin by lying flat on the ground with your legs straight up in the air at a 90-degree angle. Your arms should be straight by your sides with your palms on the ground.
2. Roll backward onto your upper back while keeping your legs straight. This will lift your butt off the ground and your feet should be roughly inline with your head.
3. Hold this position for a second and then lower yourself back to the starting position.
4. Repeat this motion as many times as you can until fatigued.

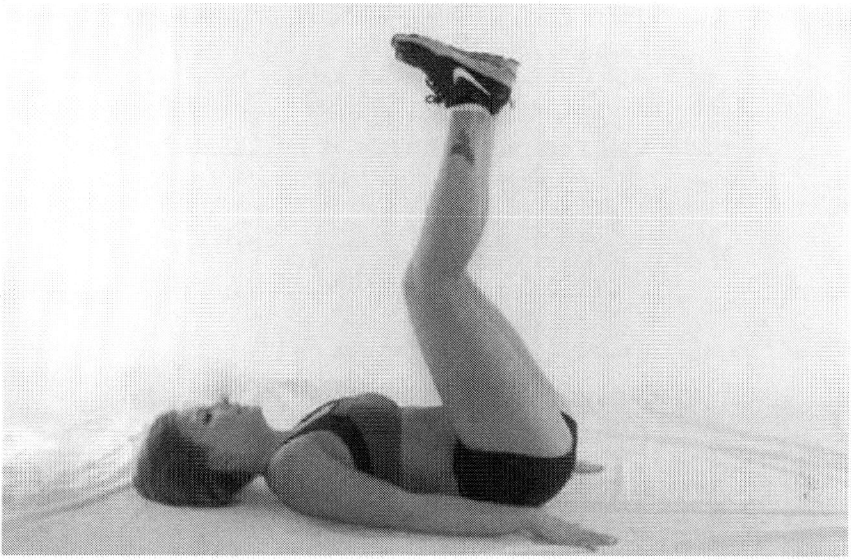

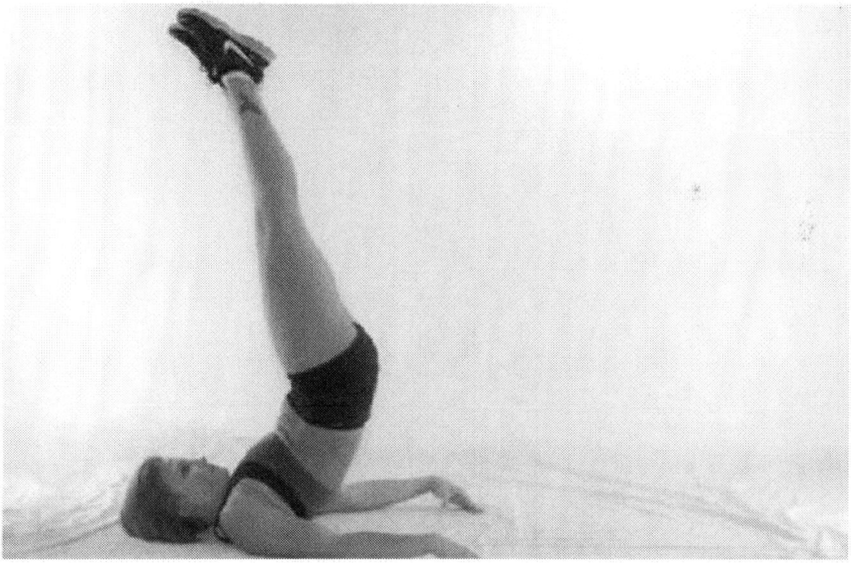

Swivel Hips

This is an advanced core training exercise that will develop and tone all of the muscles around your abdomen. It is one of the best abdominal exercises you can do.

1. Begin with your back on the ground and your knees bent with your hands palms down by your sides.
2. Lift your bent legs up by rolling your weight backward onto your upper back.
3. Swivel your hips from side to side while maintaining tension in your abs.
4. Repeat this motion until fatigued.
5. Always remember to breathe throughout the exercise. Never hold your breath.

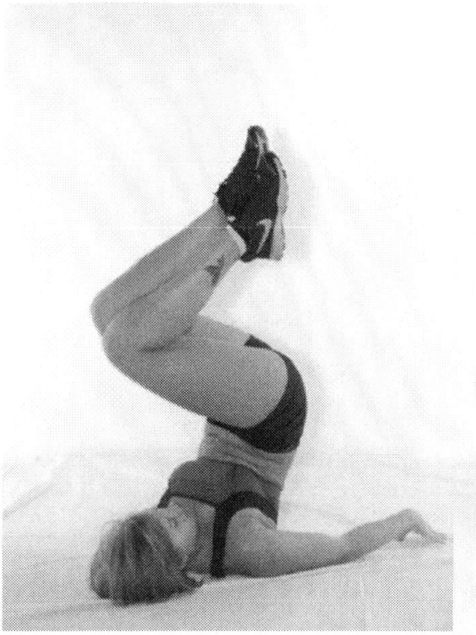

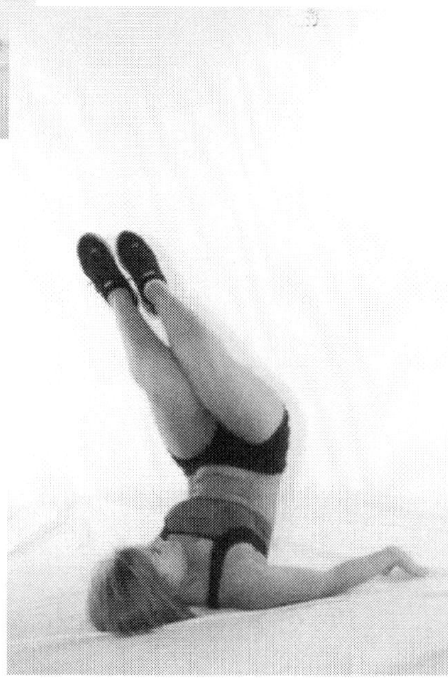

Core Training For The Side

We do not stop exercising because we grow old – we grow old because we stop exercising – Dr. Kenneth Cooper

These core training exercises are primarily focused on the muscles on the side of your waist, otherwise known as the obliques. Perform one or two of them before moving onto the core strength exercises for the back.

Oblique Curls

This core exercise looks easy but it excels at gently working your obliques.

1. Begin on all fours with your knees under your hips and your hands underneath your shoulders.

2. Tighten your ab and glute muscles to protect your lower back. This is the starting position.

3. Exhale through your mouth as you twist your right hip toward the right side of your head. Viewed from above it should look you are creating the letter C with your torso.

4. Hold for a second and then return to the starting position while you breathe in through your nose.

5. Repeat this motion on your left side.

6. Repeat this sequence 7 – 10 times or until fatigued.

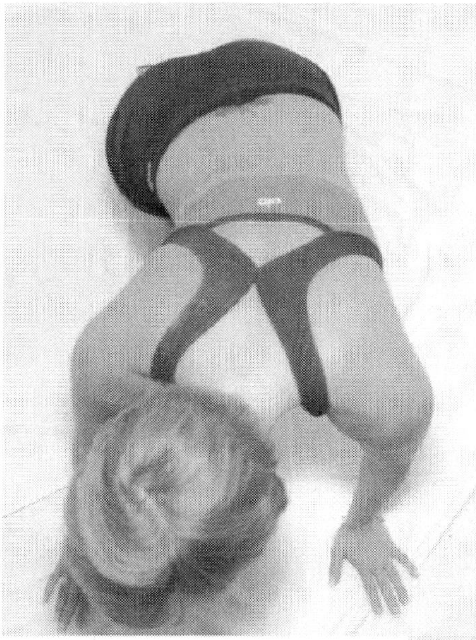

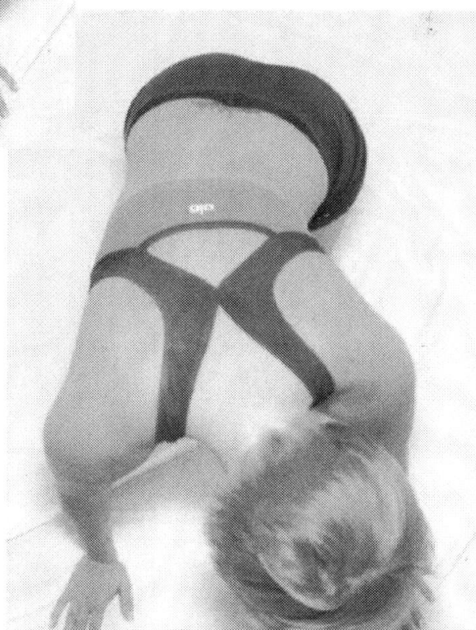

Beginners Arm Bar

The beginners arm bar is a training exercise the really focuses on the obliques while also building strength in the arms and upper body.

1. Begin by placing your right hip on the floor with your right leg extended straight out and your torso raised and supported by your right arm.

2. Place your left foot directly in front of your right knee.

3. Take a deep breath through your nose.

4. As you slowly exhale through your mouth, use your right hand and both feet to lift your hips off the ground. As you do so stretch your left arm upward as far as you can.

5. Hold this position for a slow count of five and then come down.

6. Repeat this motion for the opposite side of your body.

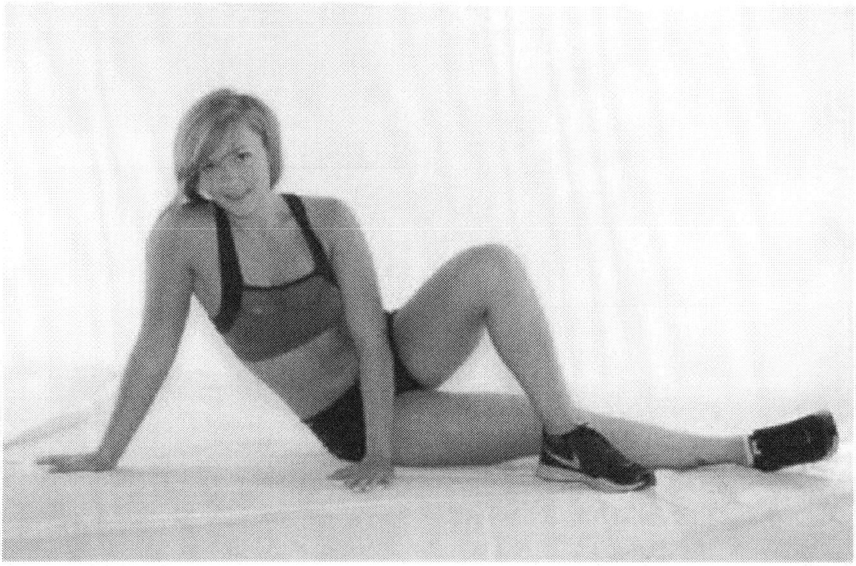

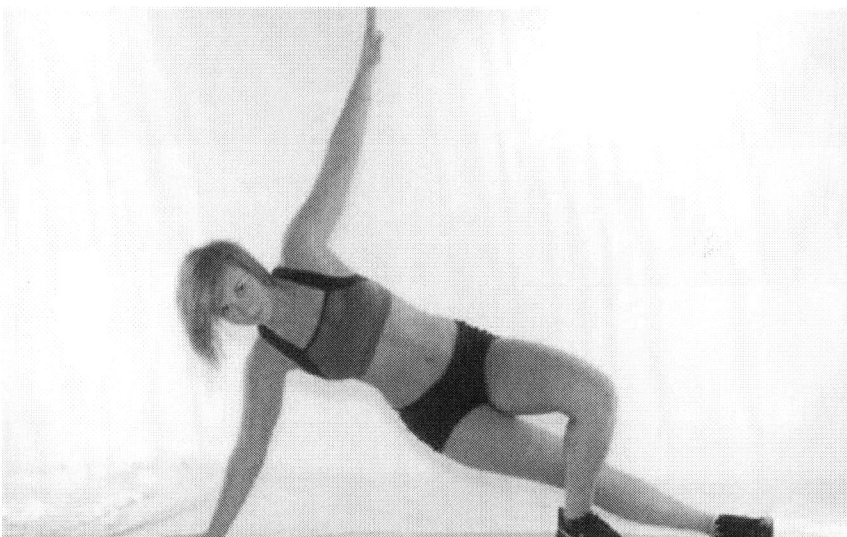

Full Arm Bar

This more advanced version of the arm bar will work your obliques even more as they will no longer be supported by your foot.

1. Begin by placing your right hip on the floor with both legs extended straight out. Your left leg should be lying directly on top of your right leg.
2. Use your right arm to prop up your torso.
3. Take a deep breath through your nose.
4. As you exhale through your mouth use your right hand and heels to lift your torso of the ground. As you do so stretch your left arm into the air as far as it will go.
5. Hold this position for a slow count of five and then lower yourself to the ground.
6. Repeat this exercise on the opposite side.

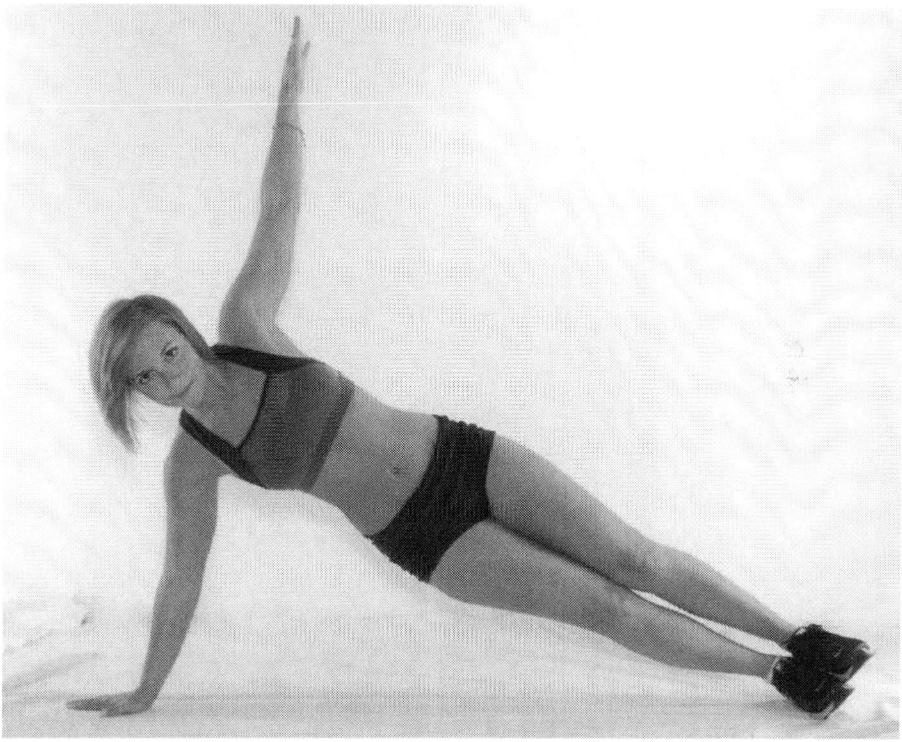

Lying Side Bends

Performing side bends on the floor provides a little more resistance than doing them standing up. If you are performing this stomach exercise on carpet, I highly recommend you wear a shirt in order to avoid rug burn.

1. Begin by lying on the floor with your knees bent and your hands behind your head.
2. Use your oblique muscles to twist your body to the side as far as you can and then the other.
3. Try for between 50 – 100 repetitions.
4. Make sure you keep your back on the floor at all times.
5. Breathe naturally throughout the exercise.

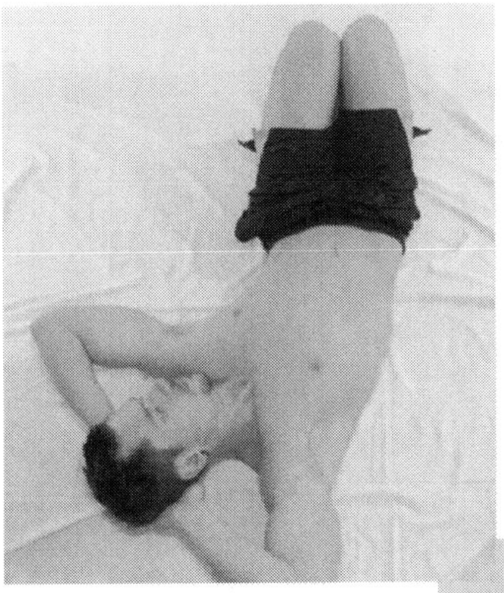

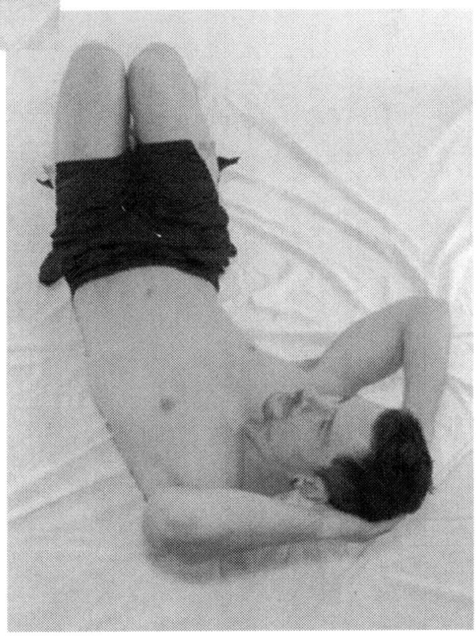

Side Bends

This core training exercise excels at strengthening and stretching your waist.

1. Begin by standing with your feet together and one arm in the air. This is the starting position.
2. Take a deep breath through your nose.
3. As you exhale through your mouth bend at the waist as far as you can go to the opposite side of your raised arm.
4. Inhale through your nose as you raise your body slightly by about five degrees. You are only moving enough to work the muscles on the side of your waist. You are not returning to the starting position.
5. Repeat this slight back and forth movement 50 to 100 times.
6. Repeat this exercise on the opposite side of your body.

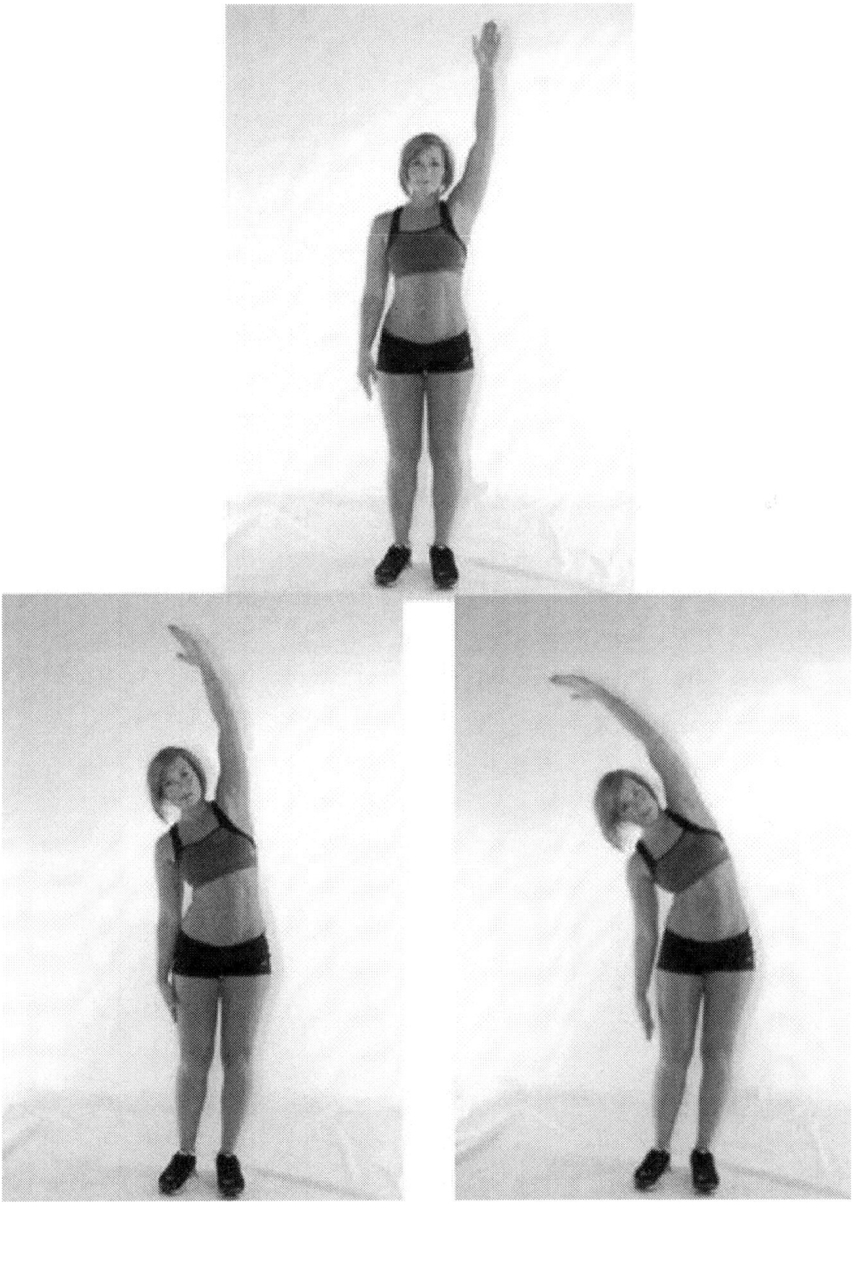

Hands Overhead Side Bends

This abdominal exercise not only works your obliques but will also expand your rib cage while strengthening your upper back and shoulders.

1. Begin with your feet shoulder width apart.

2. Interlock your fingers and reach for the ceiling with your palms facing upward. This is the starting position.

3. Inhale through your nose as you stretch to the right as far as you can go.

4. Hold this position as you exhale slowly through your mouth for 7 seconds.

5. Inhale through your nose as you return to the starting position.

6. Repeat for six repetitions and then switch sides.

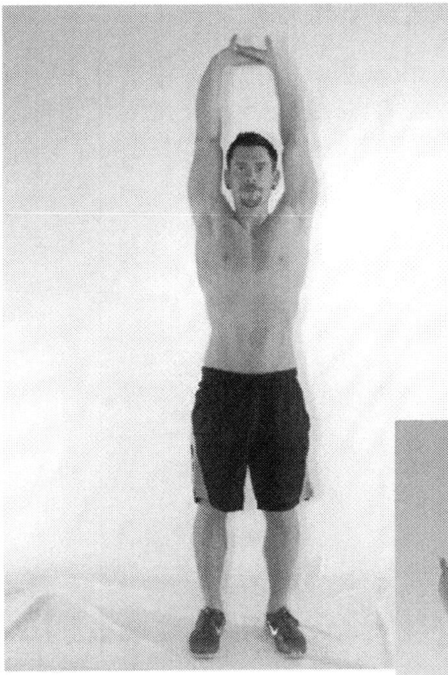

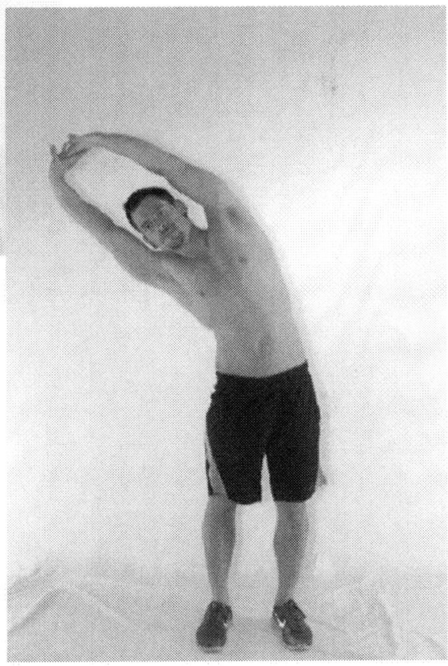

Side Ups

This abdominal exercise will not only build great core strength but also will strengthen and tone every muscle from your ankles to your shoulders.

1. Begin by lying on your right side with your right elbow directly underneath your shoulder.
2. Your upper body should be off the ground while your legs should be on it.
3. Inhale through your mouth as you straighten your body, lifting your hips off the ground.
4. Hold this position for 3 seconds and then lower yourself back to the starting position.
5. Try to perform 10 repetitions and then flip over and work the opposite side.

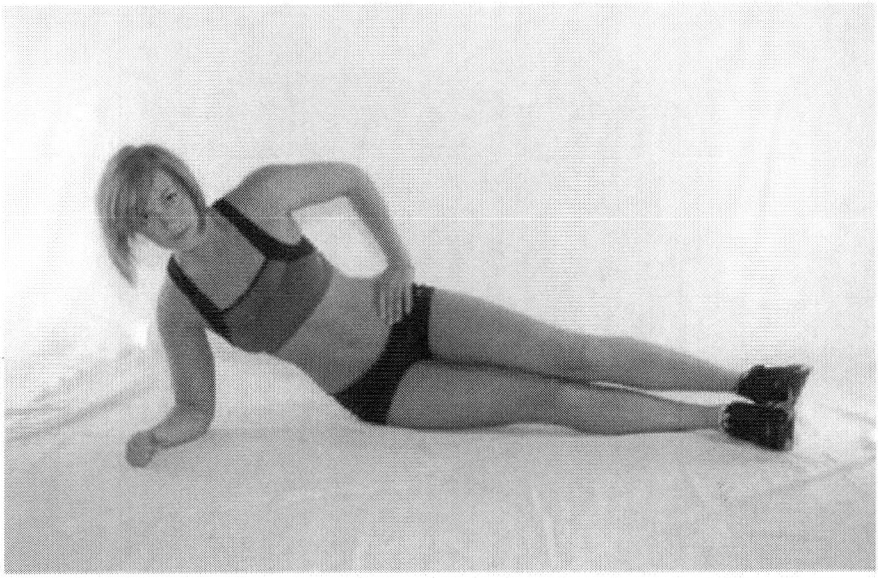

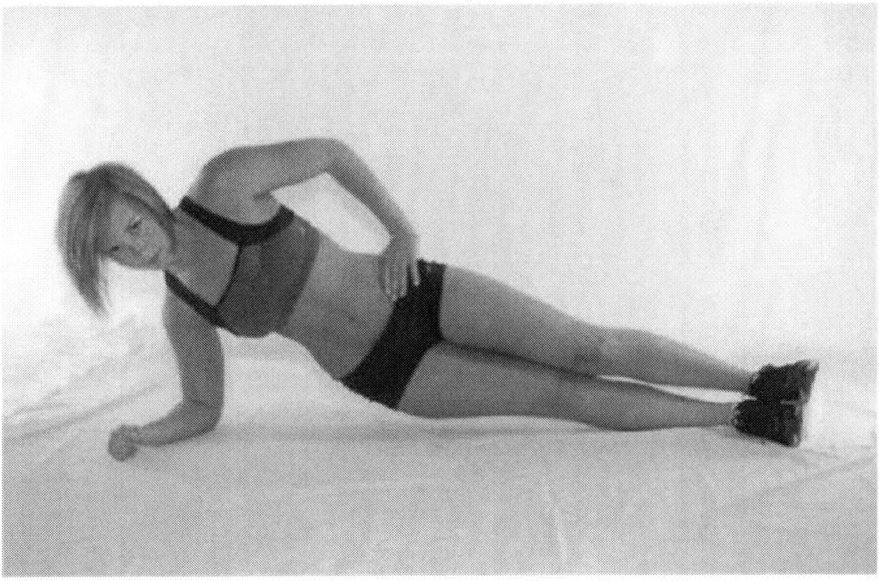

Beach Scissors

This core exercise really works your hip flexors and obliques. They are called beach scissors due to the way you prop your head up on your hand, kind of like you're lying on the beach.

1. Begin by lying on your left side with your left hand propping your head up.
2. Inhale through your nose as you raise your right leg as high as possible while keeping it straight.
3. Hold for 3 seconds and then return to the starting position. Repeat this motion until fatigued.
4. Flip over and repeat on the opposite side.

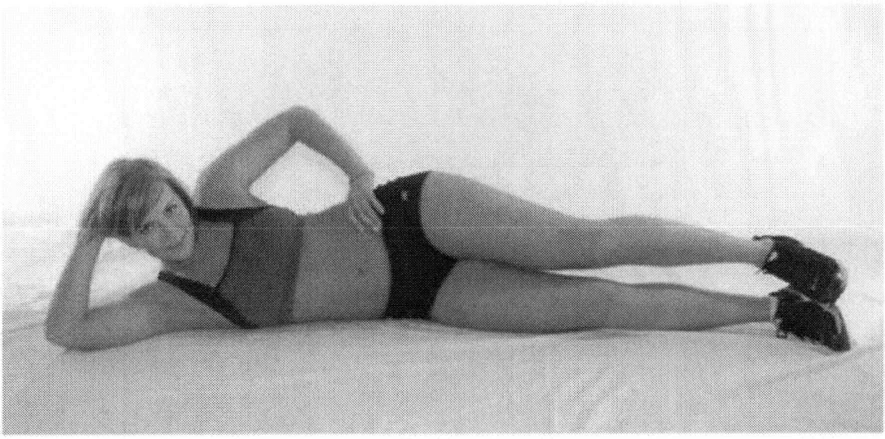

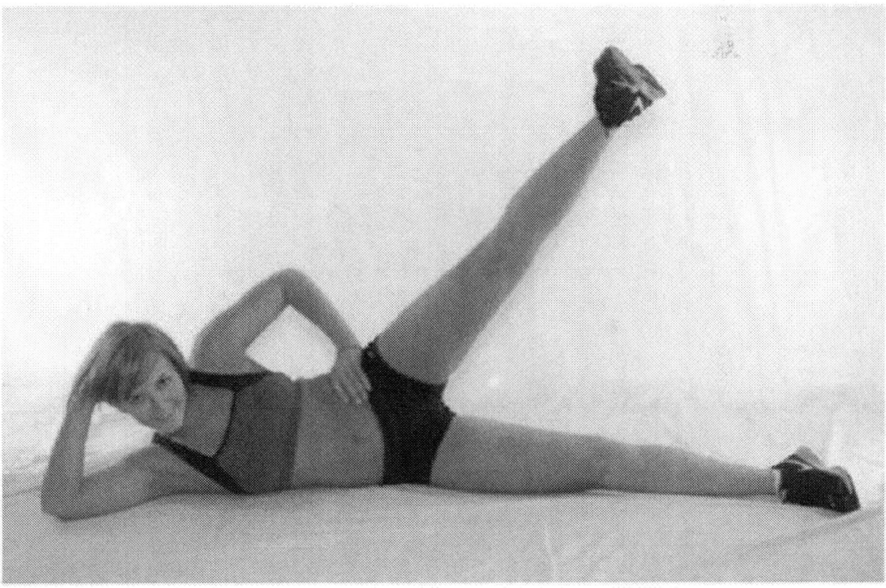

Advanced Beach Scissors

This core strength exercise combines a side plank with a scissors motion. This is a great core training exercise as it works all of your core muscles, especially your abdomen.

1. Begin by resting on your left side with your elbow holding yourself up. Your whole body should be as straight as a board.
2. Keep your stomach and butt muscles tight.
3. Inhale through your nose and then raise your right leg while keeping it straight.
4. Hold your right leg for 3 seconds in the raised position before lowering it.
5. Repeat until fatigued.
6. Flip over and perform the exercise again with your left leg.

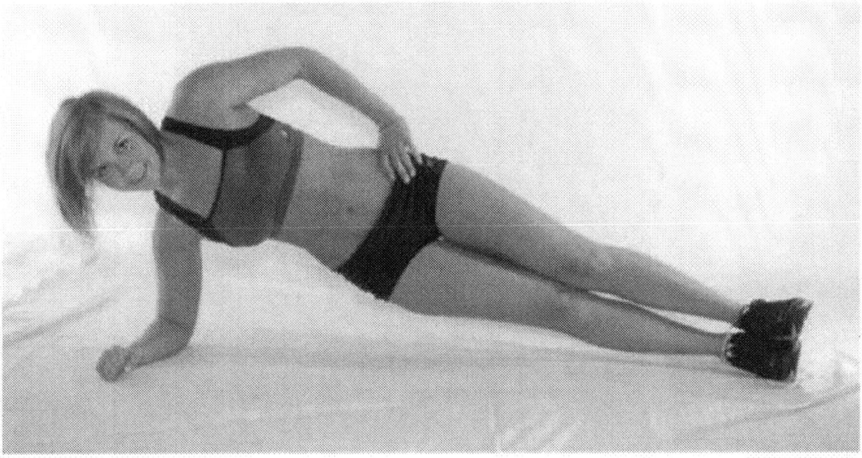

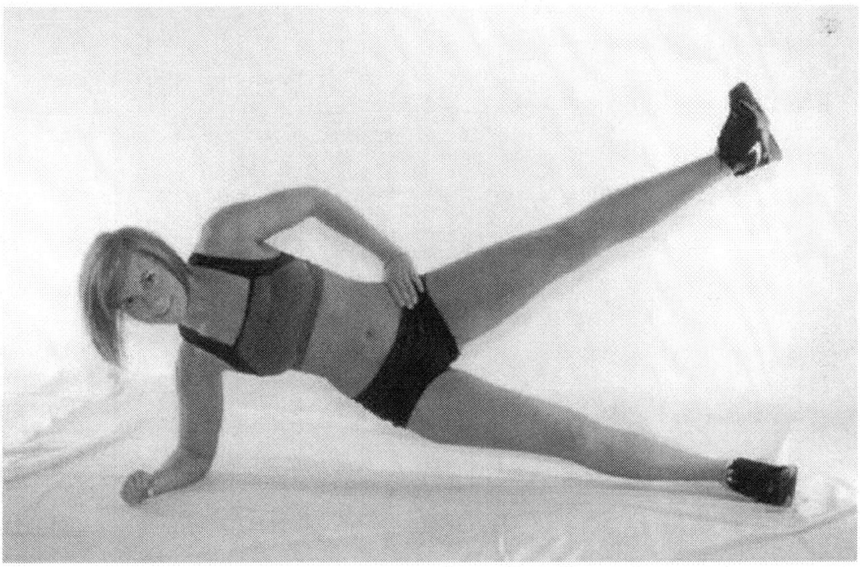

Sideward Leg Lifts

Sideward leg lifts will help you develop flexibility and strength in your hips and thighs.

1. Begin by lying on your side with your legs together.
2. Lift both legs off the ground at the same time. Inhale through your nose as you lift them up, exhale as you lower them to the floor.
3. Repeat until fatigued and then switch sides.

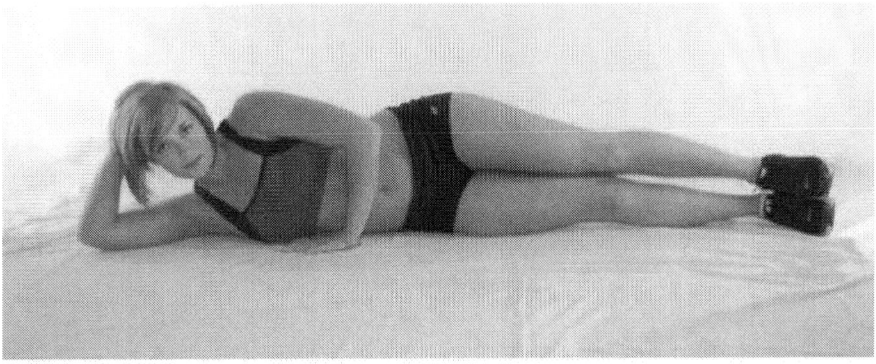

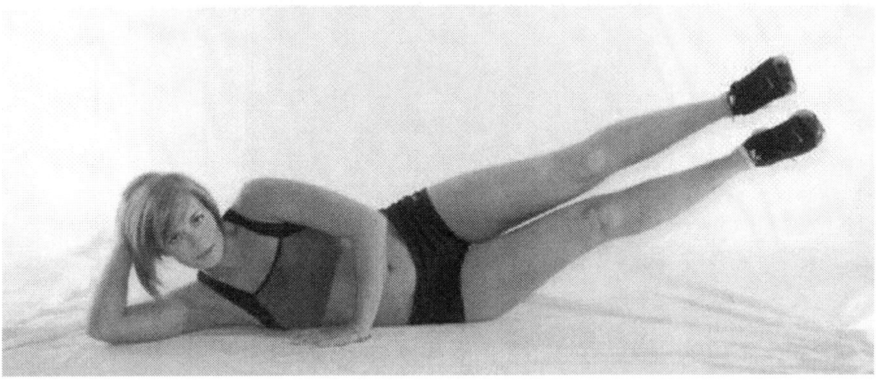

Iron Crosses

This ab exercise is not easy but it will build incredible core strength by making your abs, obliques and intercostal muscles burn. If you find it too difficult at first bending your knees will reduce the leverage and make it easier.

1. Begin by lying flat on your back with your legs straight up in the air and your arms by your side for support. Your legs should make a 90-degree angle with your body.
2. Lift your head slightly off the ground. This will help protect and strengthen your neck.
3. Inhale through your nose as you lower your legs to the right as far as you can without touching the ground. From above your body should look like a big L.
4. Exhale through your mouth as you raise your legs back to the starting position.
5. Inhale through your nose again and lower your legs to the left side as far as you can without touching the floor.
6. Exhale through your mouth and raise your legs back up to the starting position.
7. Do as many as you can until fatigued.

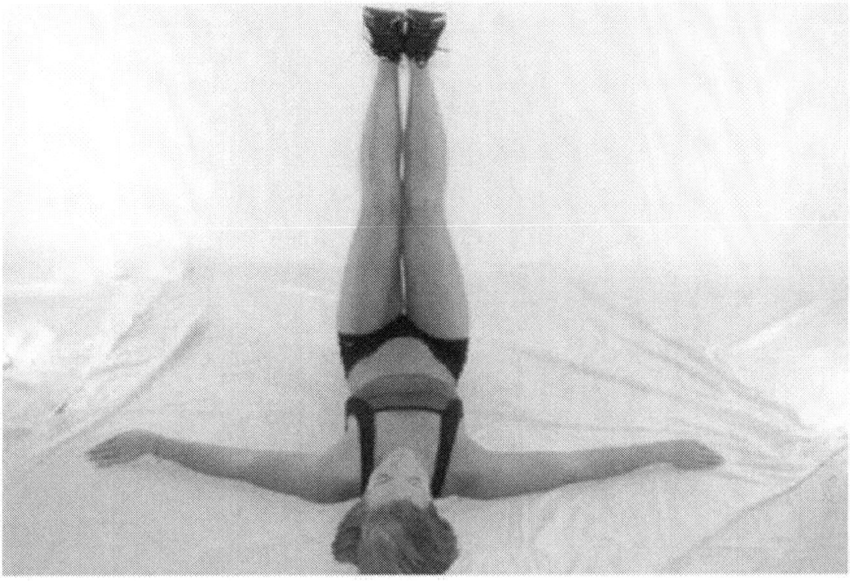

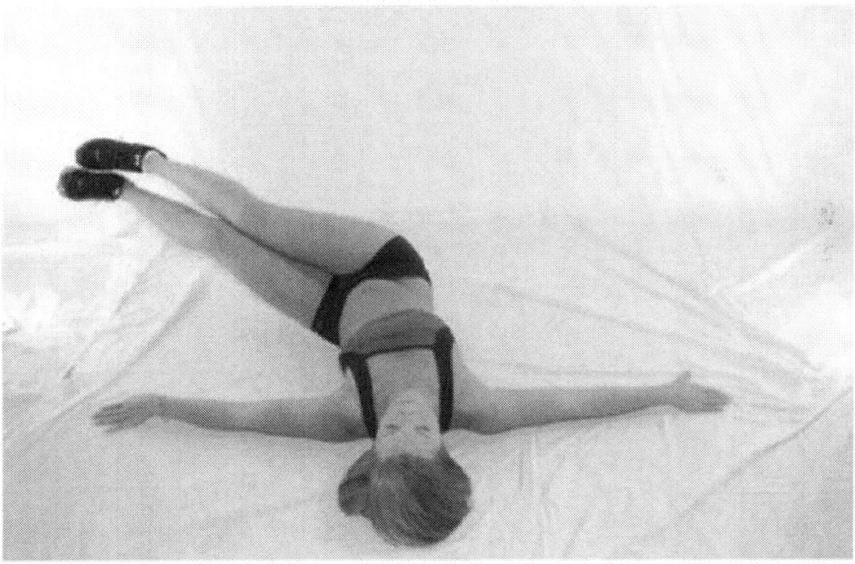

Grounded Bicycles

This is one of the best abdominal exercises you can do if you want a flat belly. It will really hit your abs, intercostal muscles and obliques.

1. Begin by lying flat on your back with your legs straight and your hands behind your head.
2. Lift both your legs about six inches off the ground.
3. Lift your head off the ground.
4. Bring your right knee toward your chest and try and meet it with your left elbow.
5. Straighten your right leg and then bend your left knee toward your right elbow.
6. Keep your abs tight and remember to breathe at all times.
7. Try doing 10 in a row in a slow and controlled manner.

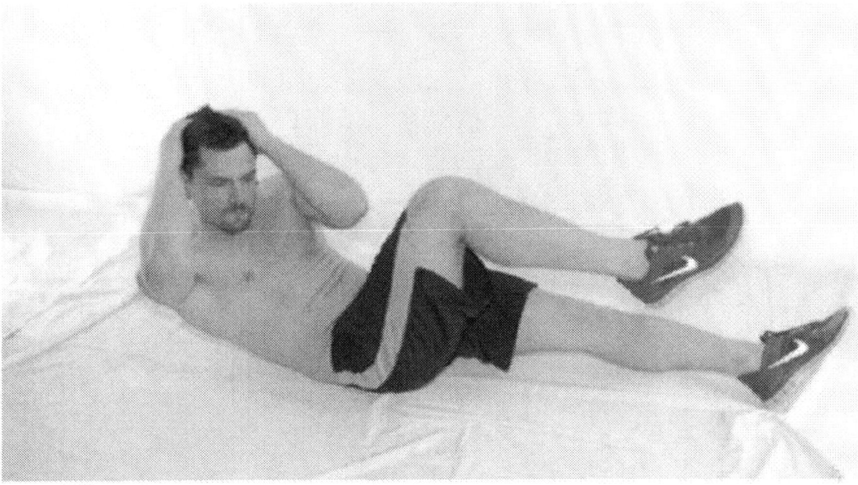

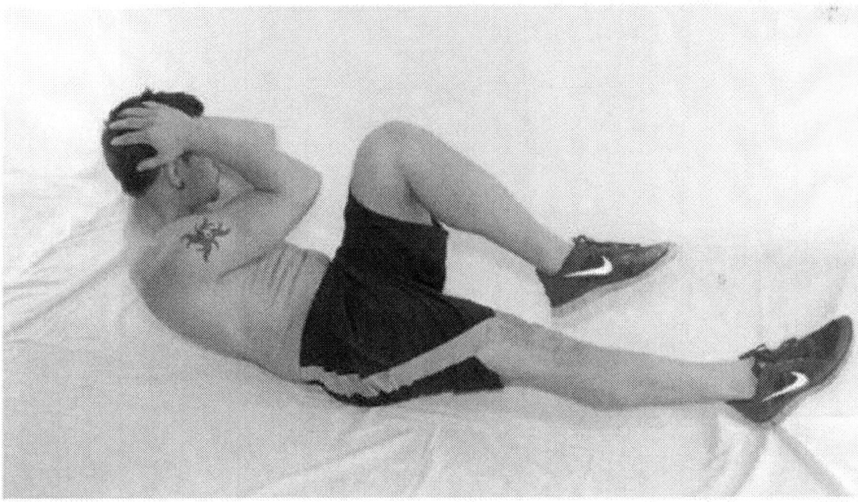

Russian Twists

This ab exercise really hits your entire core region as both your upper and lower body are off the ground. The twisting motion will really strengthen your obliques, as well as, help with the suppleness of your spine.

1. Begin by sitting up on the ground with your feet raised in front of you.
2. Fold your arms across your chest and then begin to twist at your torso from left to right.
3. Make sure you keep your feet off the ground at all times.
4. Do as many twists as you can until fatigued.

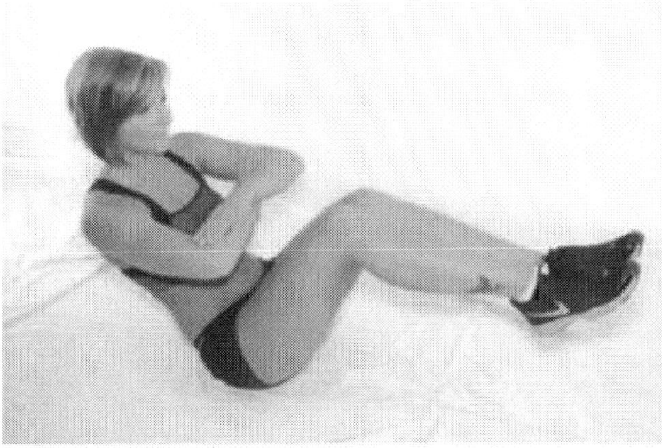

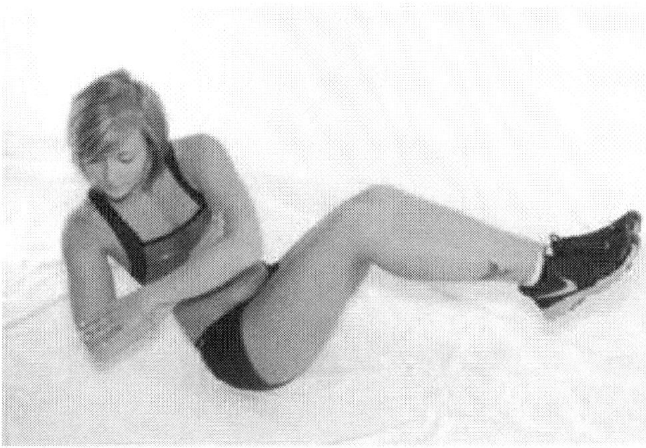

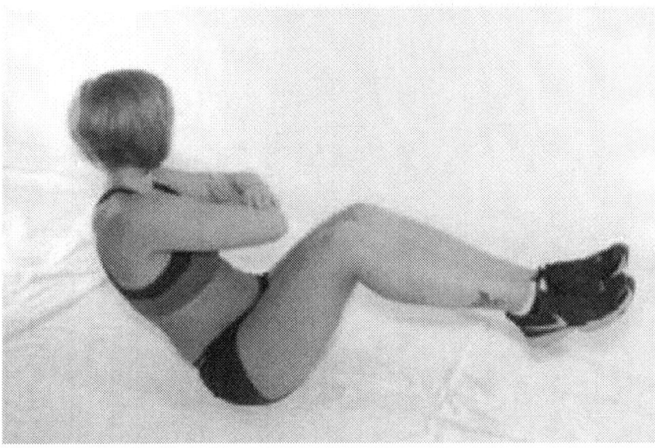

Core Exercises For The Back

Strive for progress, not perfection. –Unknown

If we're going to work the core muscles in the front and side it only makes sense to work the back muscles as well. Most of these exercises involve some form of back bending, as this is the best way to work the back and spine. Again, pick one or two of these exercises. The easier ones are at the beginning and they increase in difficulty from there.

Ying/Yang Bends

For many of you this may be your first introduction to a back bending exercise. The key is to move slowly and deliberately while keeping your abs tight at all times, particularly for the forward bends. Keep your knees slightly bent as this takes pressure off your lower back.

1. With your feet shoulder width apart and your knees slightly bent, place your hands on your lower back.
2. Breathe in through your nose as you bend your back backward, almost as if you are trying to look at the ceiling. Go as far as you can while maintaining your balance.
3. Exhale through your mouth as you bend forward at your waist trying to touch your hands to the floor. If you can't reach the floor or if your back is tight, feel free to increase the bend in your knees.
4. Repeat this motion 10 times.

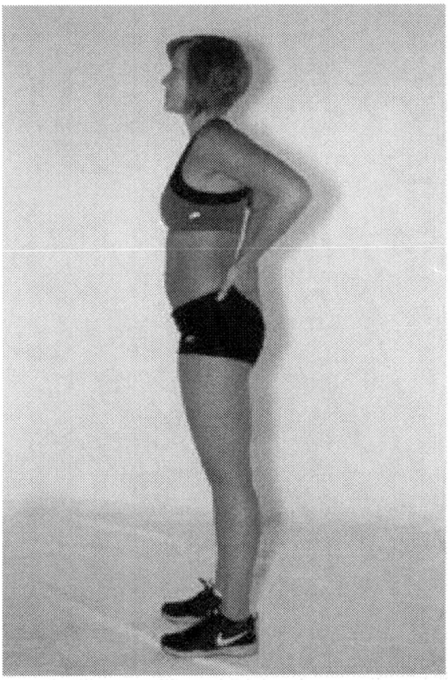

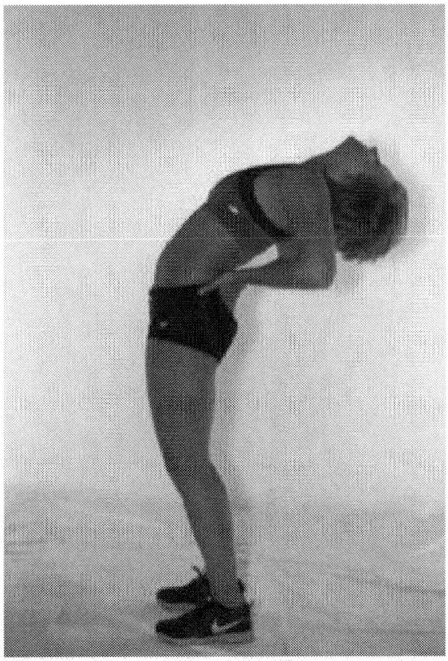

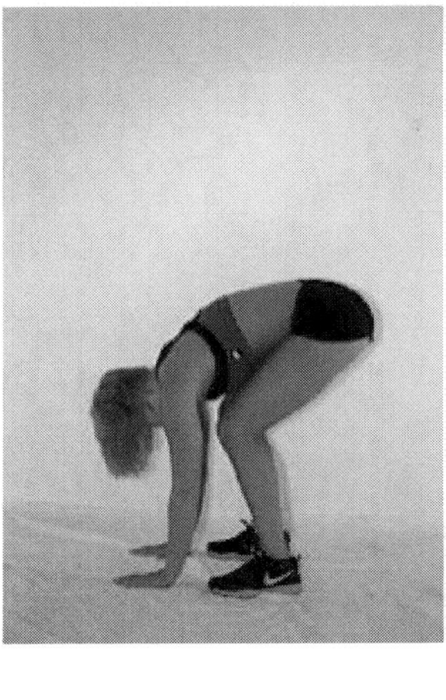

Kneeling Back Arch

This core training exercise not only works your back but your abs and butt as well.

1. Kneel on the floor with your arms and thighs at a 90-degree angle to your body.
2. Exhale through your mouth as you look up while allowing your back to curve downward. Hold this position for a count of 10.
3. Inhale through your mouth as you allow your head to fall forward while arching your back upward. Hold for another count of 10.
4. Perform this movement slowly and deliberately while ensuring that your weight is evenly distributed between your knees and hands.
5. Repeat this movement 10 times.

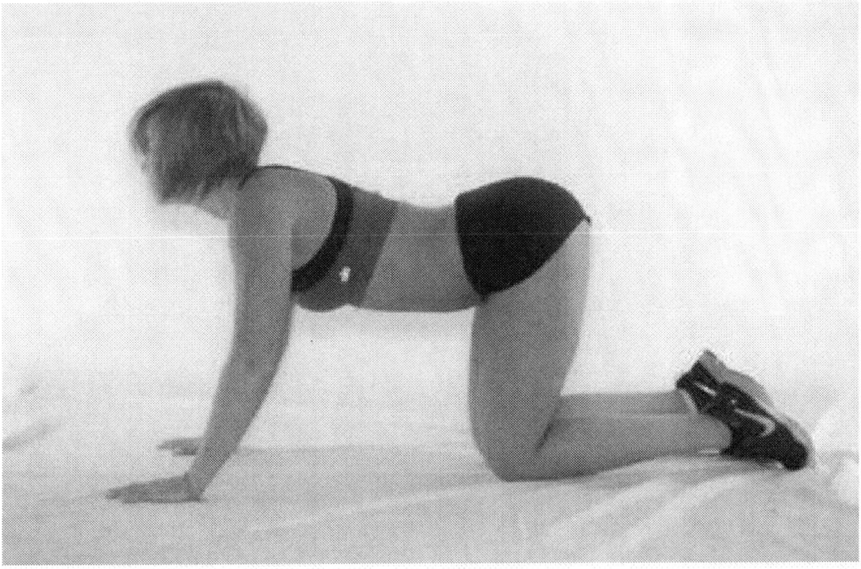

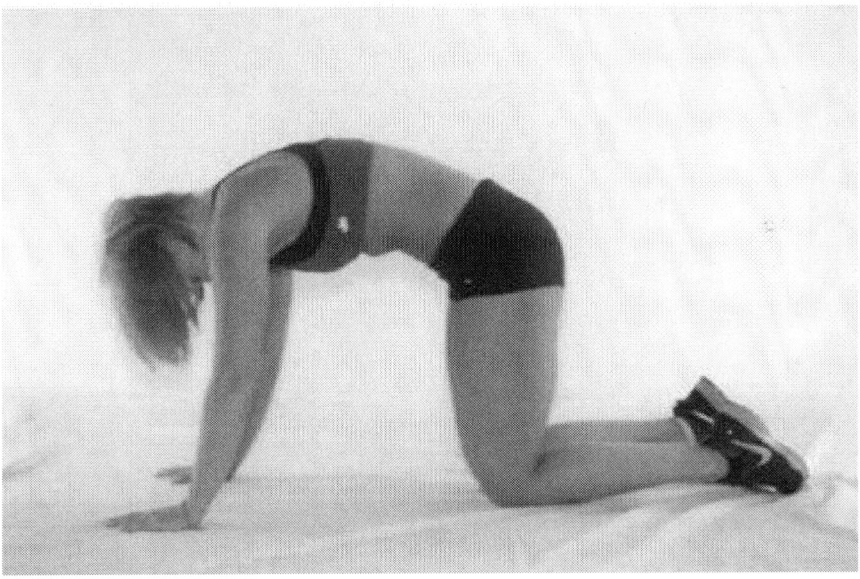

Cobra Pushup

The cobra pushup is a variation of the cobra pose that is commonly done in yoga. Although it is called a pushup, the primary muscles you want to use are those in your lower back. Your arms are only to be used for support.

1. Lie flat on your stomach with your hands by your chest.
2. Tighten your abs and breathe in through your nose as you use your lower back muscles to lift your chest off the ground. Go as high as you are comfortable going. Use your arms only as support. The goal here is to strengthen your lower back.
3. At the highest point, breathe out through your mouth as you hold this position for a count of 5.
4. Breathe in through your nose as you lower yourself to the ground.
5. Perform 15 repetitions.

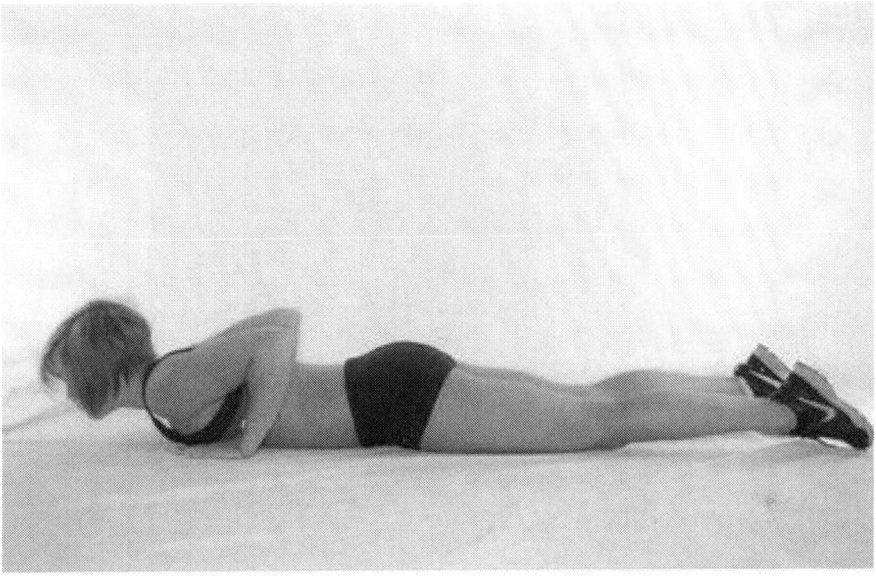

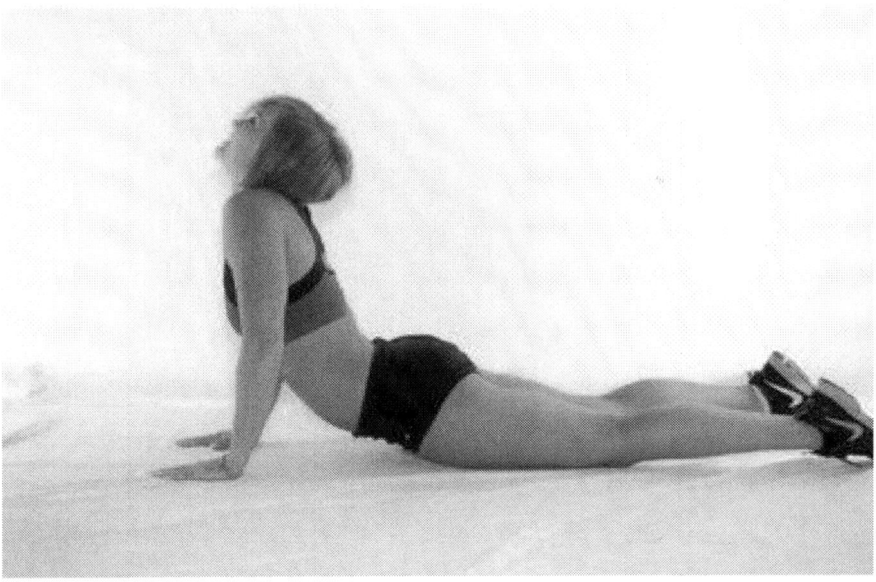

Easy Bridge

If you are a beginner to bridging, this is a good place to start. It remains an excellent core exercise although it doesn't work your neck.

1. Begin by lying on the floor with your knees bent and your feet flat on the floor.
2. Place your arms straight beside you with your palms on the ground.
3. Inhale through your nose as you use your core strength to lift your hips toward the ceiling.
4. Exhale through your mouth as you hold this position for 7 seconds.
5. Lower yourself to the floor.
6. Repeat this exercise 5 – 8 times.

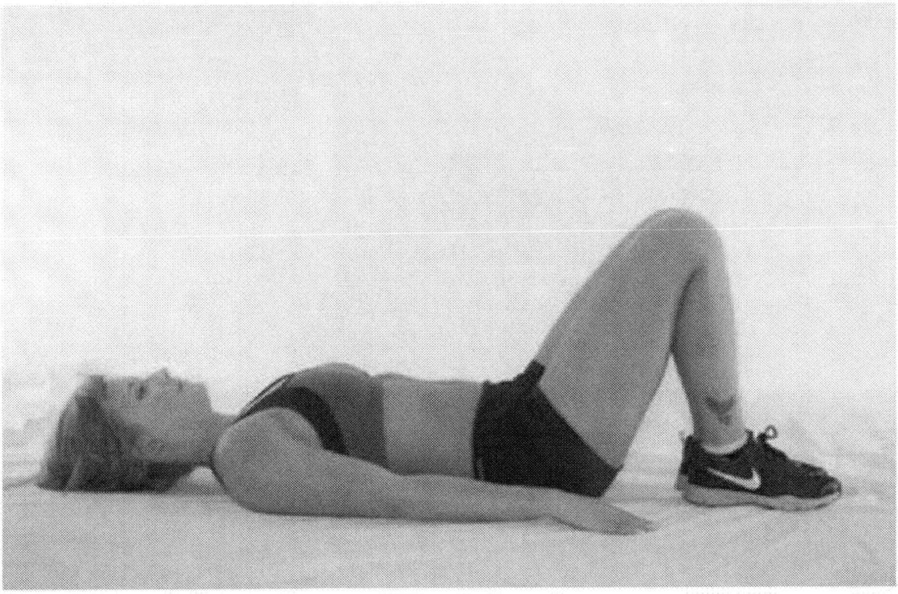

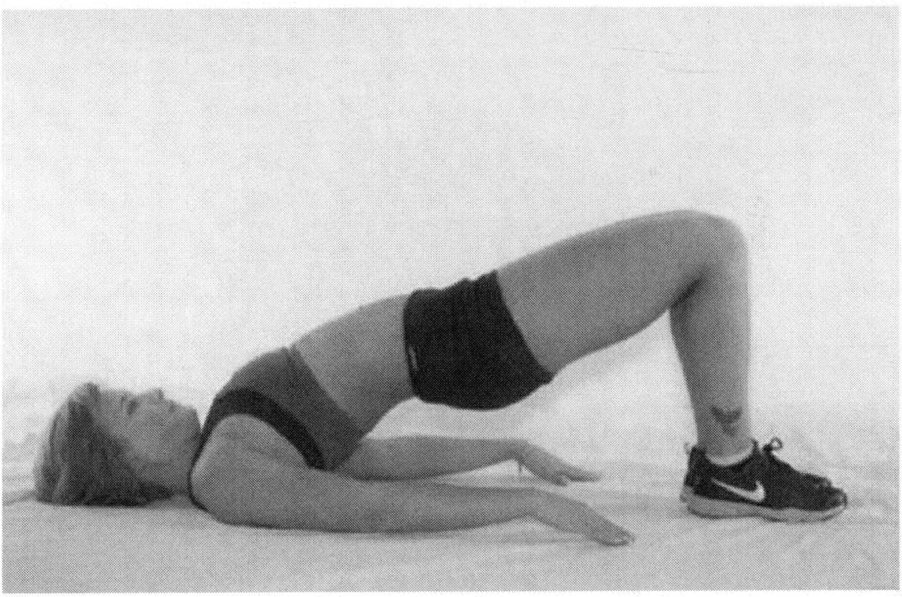

Single Leg Easy Bridge

This is a slightly more advanced version of the easy bridge. Using only one leg forces your core to work extra hard to maintain your balance which is useful if you desire a flat belly.

1. Begin by lying on the floor with your knees bent and your feet flat on the floor.
2. Place your arms straight beside you with your palms on the ground.
3. Place your right ankle just below your left knee.
4. Inhale through your nose as you use your core strength to lift your hips toward the ceiling.
5. Exhale through your mouth as you hold this position for 7 seconds.
6. Lower yourself to the floor.
7. Repeat this exercise 5 times.
8. Repeat this exercise with your left ankle over your right knee.

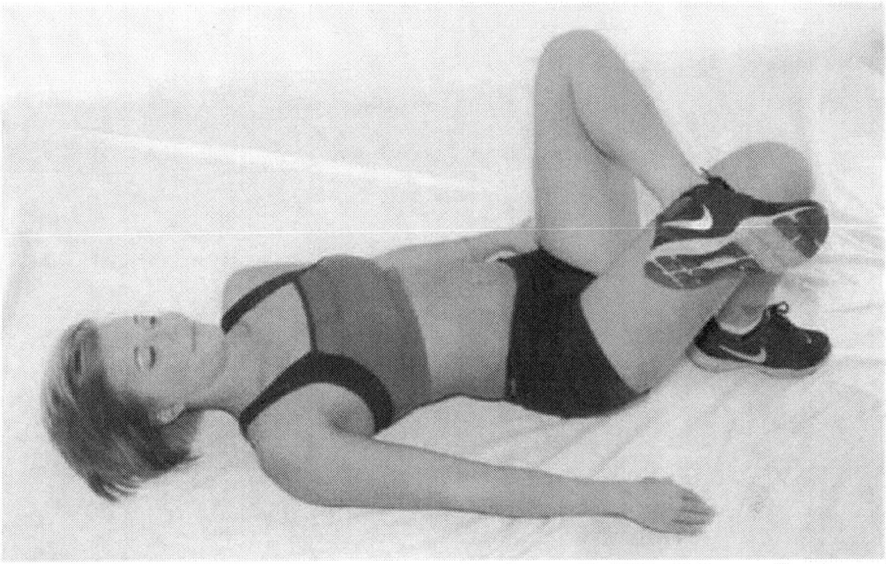

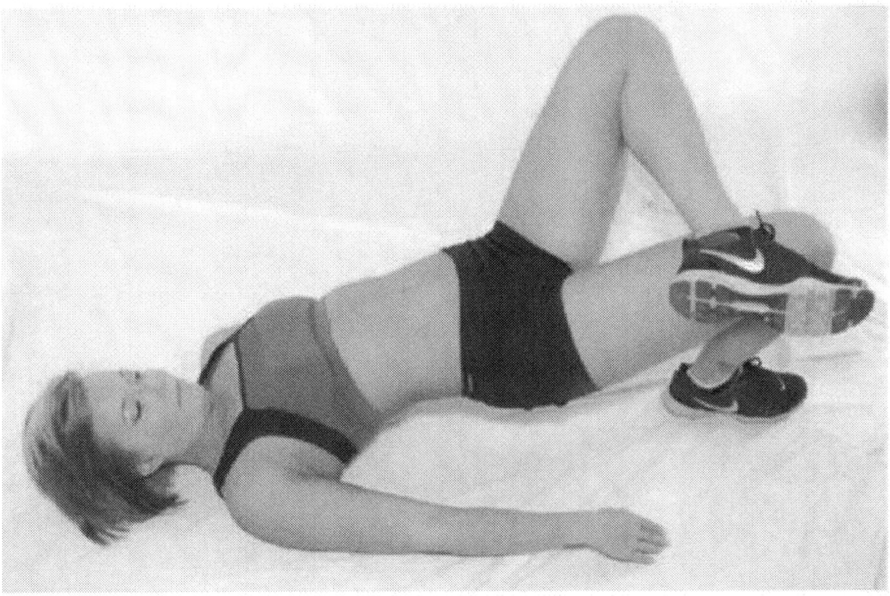

Plank

Planks may be one of the most popular core exercises of recent years. The reason for this is that not only does planking work your core but it also hits every muscle from your shoulders to your calves.

1. Begin with your stomach on the floor.
2. Prop yourself up on your elbows. Try to place your elbows directly below your shoulders.
3. Now simply breathe in through your nose and exhale through your mouth as you try to hold this position for as long as you can. When you can hold this position for 2 minutes, you are doing well.

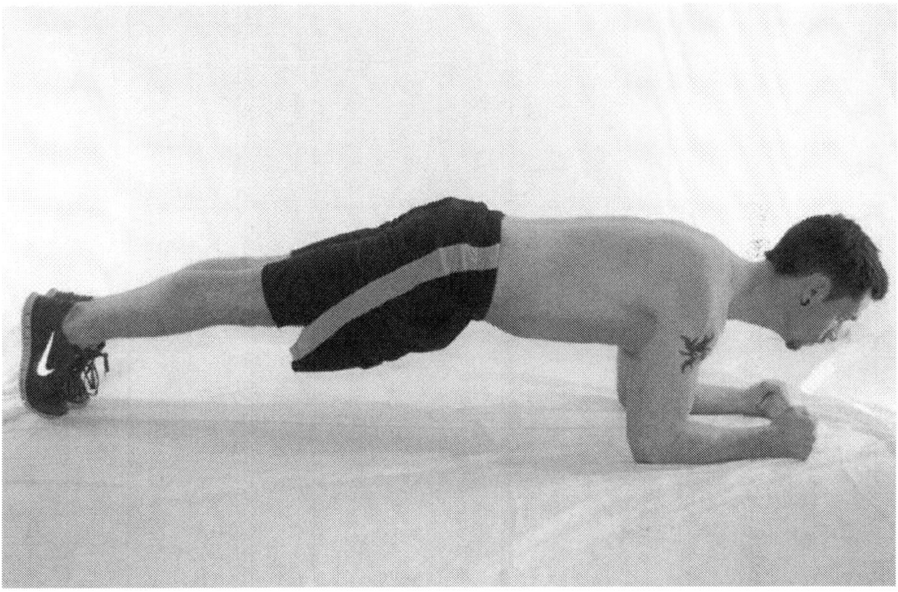

Reverse Leg Lifts

This ab exercise stretches and strengthens your lower back while at the same time working your abdominals and glutes. When you lift your legs it is very important to keep your nose on the floor in order to protect your lower back.

1. Begin by lying flat on the floor face down with your arms stretched forward.
2. Inhale through your nose and use your back muscles to lift both of your legs at the same time. Try and hold this position for a count of 5.
3. Exhale through your mouth and slowly lower your legs to the floor.
4. Repeat this movement 10 times.

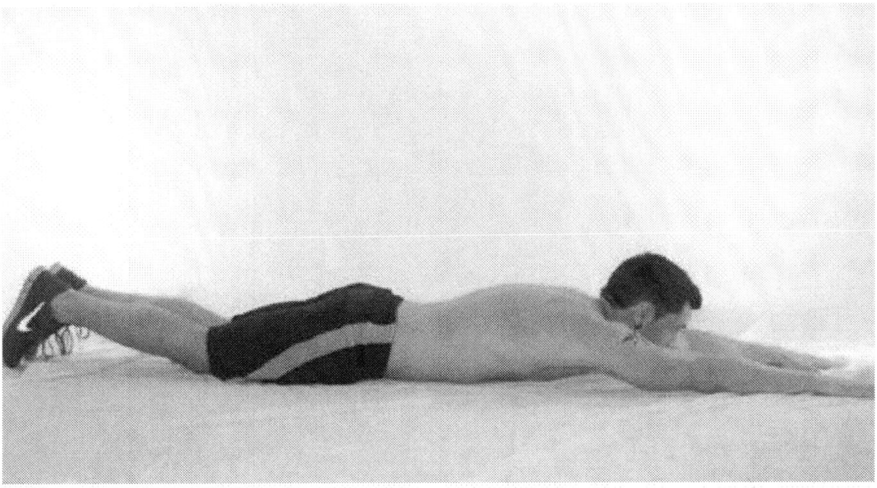

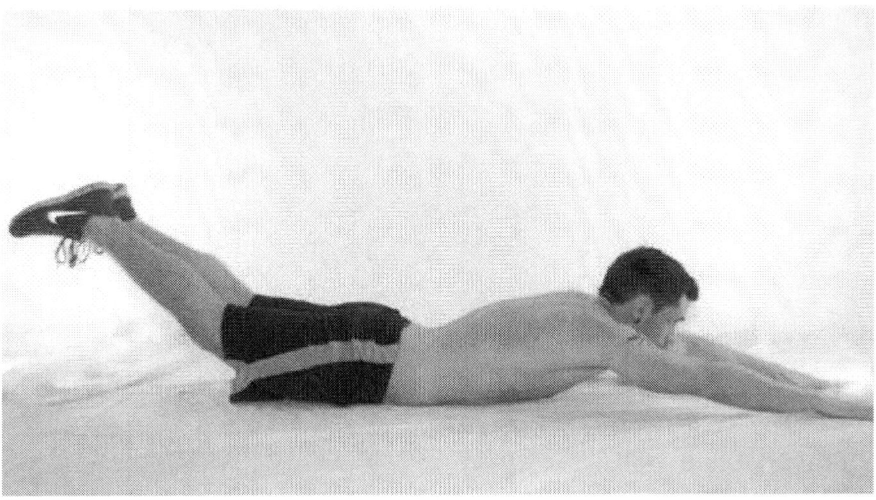

Torso Lifts

Torso lifts are the opposite of the reverse leg lifts although they still work your back and abdominals.

1. Lie face down on the floor with your arms stretched forward.
2. Inhale through your nose filling your lungs.
3. Exhale through your mouth as you lift your arms, chest and abdominals as high as can. Keep your legs on the ground at all times while squeezing your butt to protect your lower back. Hold this position for a count of 5.
4. Lower yourself to the floor and inhale through your nose.
5. Repeat this exercise 10 times or until fatigued.

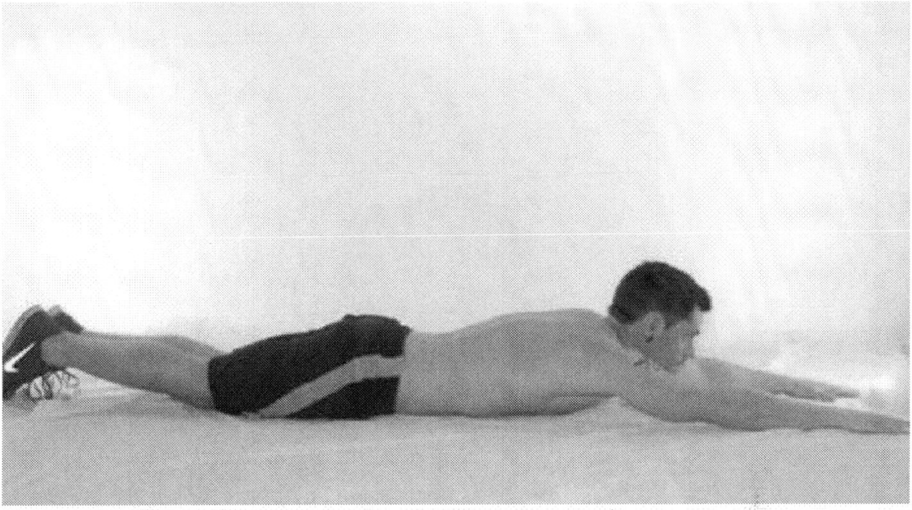

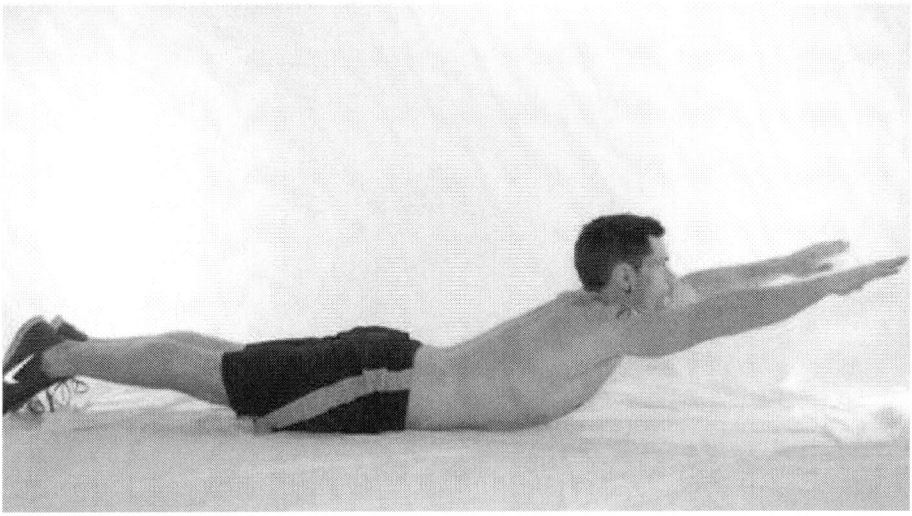

Arch Ups

This core exercise combines the torso lift and reverse leg exercises. It is excellent for developing a strong back, shoulders, legs and glutes while increasing your flexibility.

1. Begin by lying on your stomach with your arms shoulder width apart and your legs together.
2. Stretch your body lengthwise.
3. Tighten your butt and abdominal muscles as you arch your back, lifting your arms and legs off the ground as you do so.
4. When you've arched your back as far as it will go hold this position for a count of two while keeping your arms by your ears. Your body should be shaped liked the bottom of a rocker on a rocking chair.
5. Lower yourself back to the starting position.
6. Do as many as you can until fatigued. When you can do 25 in a row you are doing well.

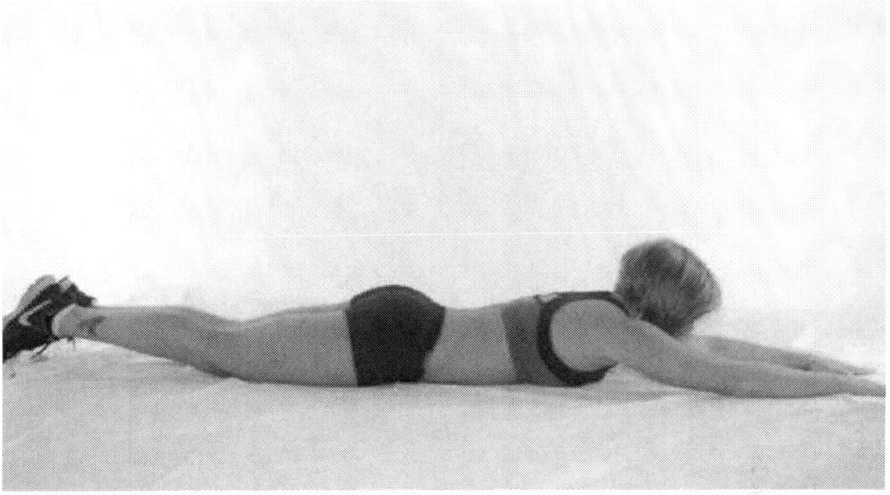

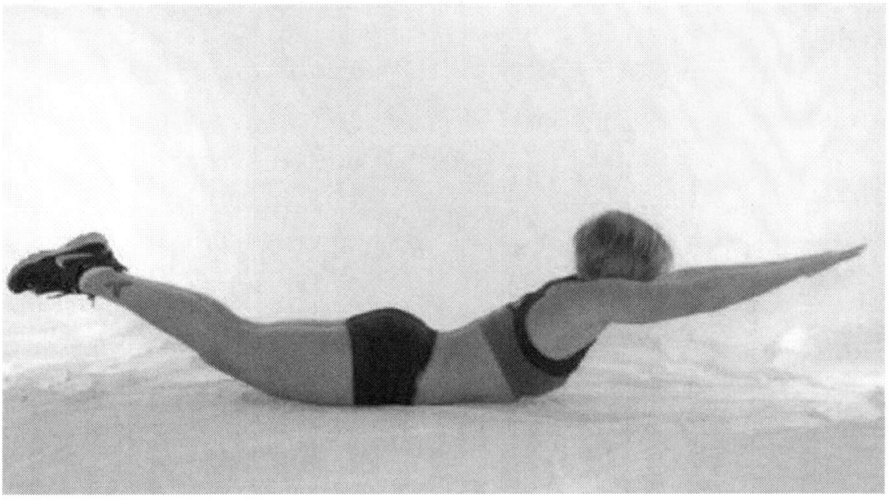

Tight Arch Rocks

This core training exercise will have you rocking back and forth like the bottom of a rocking chair. This motion will strengthen and lengthen your entire body while tightening your butt, legs and abs. Aside from gaining a flat belly, this exercise will also increase the flexibility of your abs and lower back.

1. Begin by lying on your belly on the ground. Tighten your abs and glutes as you raise both your legs and arms into the air.
2. Begin to rock back and forth like a rocker on the bottom of a rocking chair. Keep all of your muscles tight and point your toes.
3. Breathe deeply through your nose and mouth at all times. Never hold your breath.
4. Maintain a strong arched position as you continue rocking for 15 repetitions or until fatigued.

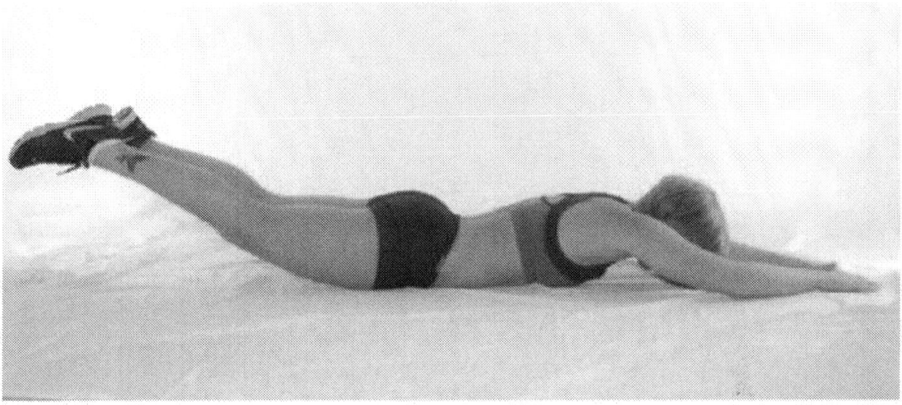

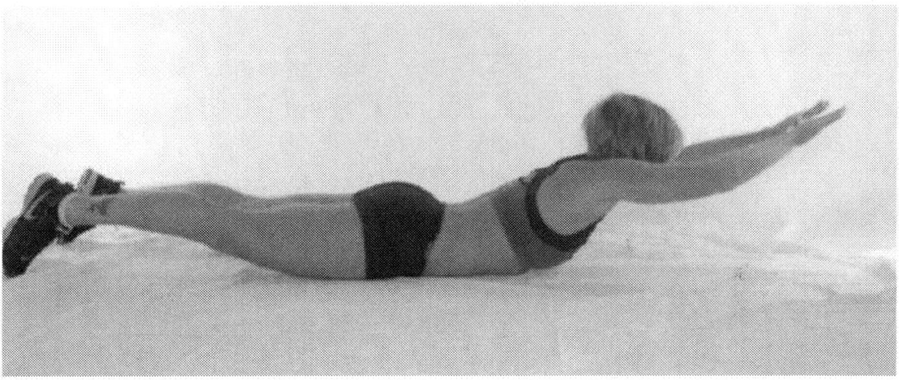

Swimmers

This exercise is fantastic for strengthening your back while simultaneously sculpting your glutes.

1. Begin by lying flat down on your stomach with your arms in front of you.
2. Slowly raise your right leg and your left arm as high as possible.
3. Hold this position at its highest point for 3 seconds.
4. Lower your arm and leg to the ground and then repeat with your opposite arm and leg.
5. Switch back and forth in this manner until fatigued. When you can do 10 in a row you are doing well.

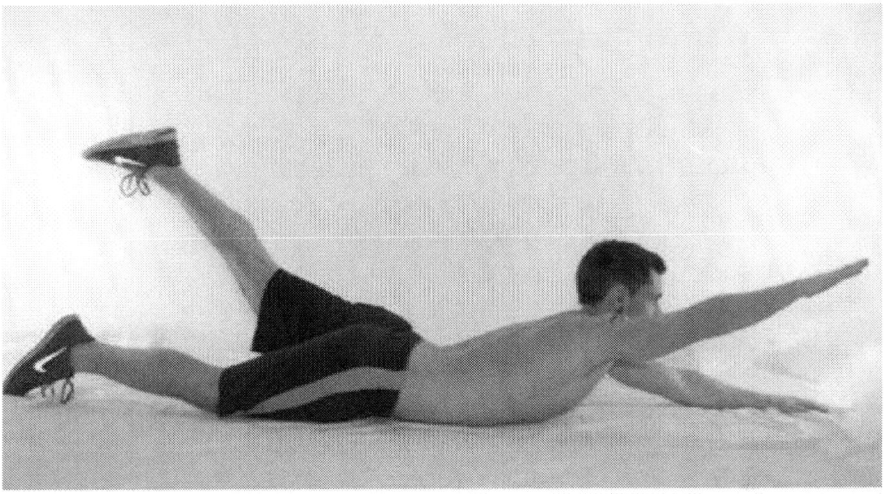

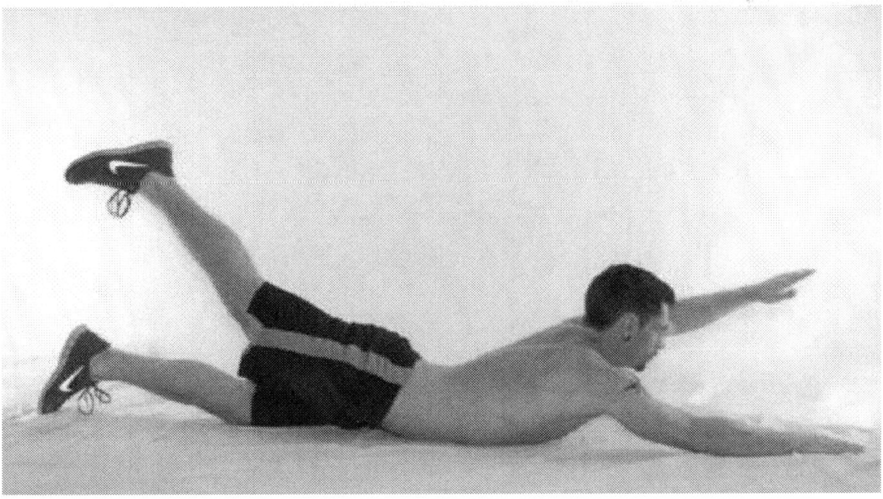

Floor Bow Posture

This posture is commonly practiced in yoga. It is fantastic at increasing the flexibility of your spine while stretching and strengthening the muscles, as well. When I perform the floor bow, I generally get the best results doing it twice. You can do more if you feel your back needs it.

1. Begin by lying flat on your stomach.
2. Grab your ankles from the outside with either hand.
3. Use your legs to kick up and backward. All of the force should be generated by your legs, not your arms. Your arms should be like ropes. They are attached to your ankles, but they are not generating any pulling force themselves.
4. If you are able, try to look at the ceiling by bending your neck backward. If your neck is stiff, simply bend it backward as far as you can.
5. Hold this position while taking five slow, deep breaths.

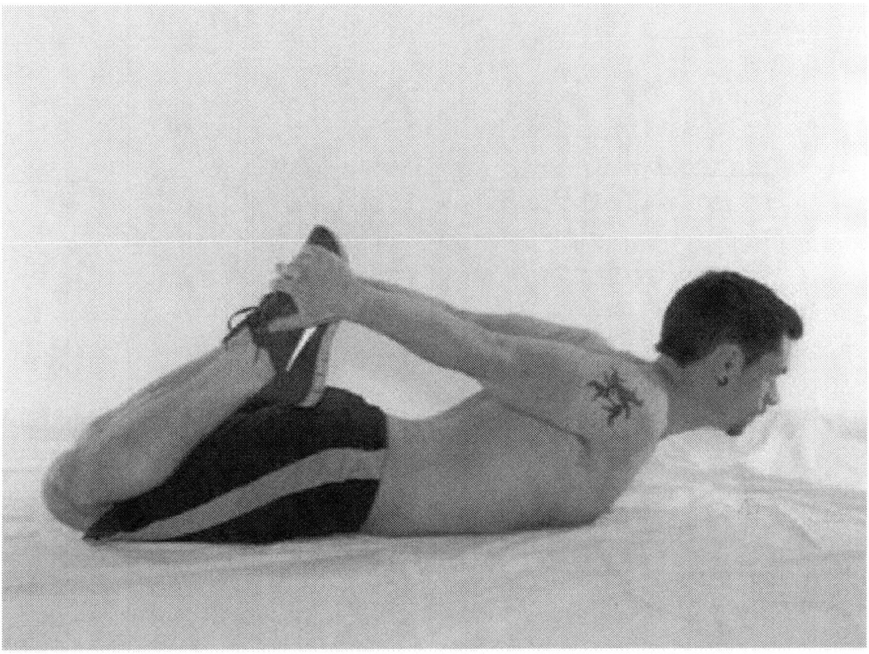

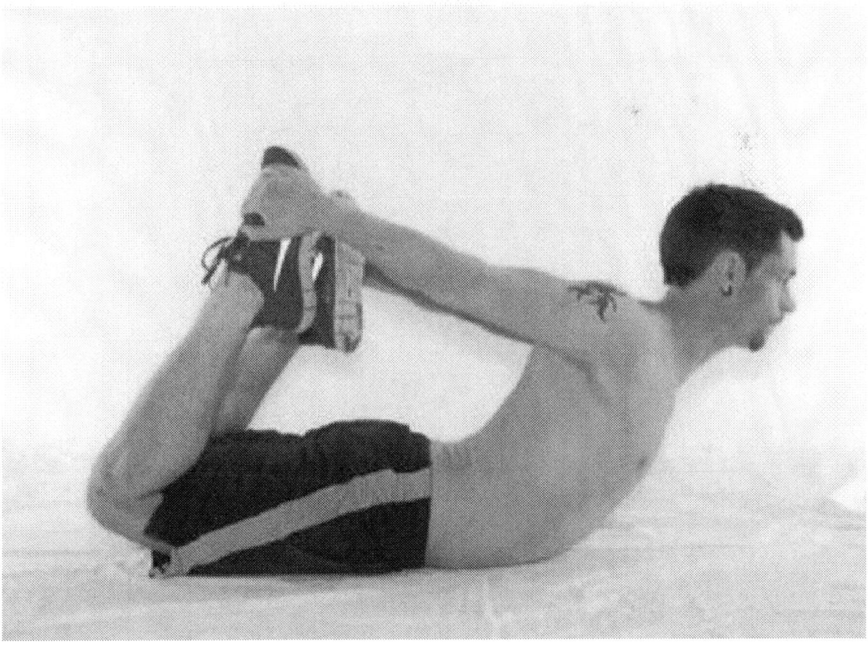

Flying Plank

This ab exercise will not only help you get a flat belly and a strong core, but will work your pectorals, triceps and deltoids as well. Once again the fact that this exercise forces you to keep your balance will work your muscles in a way that is simply impossible on a machine.

1. Begin in the classic pushup position. Tense your butt and ab muscles to support your lower back.
2. Raise your right leg straight behind you as far as you can while you raise your left arm so that it is parallel to your body.
3. Breathe in through your nose and out through your mouth. Hold this position as long as you can. Lower your leg and arm to the ground.
4. Repeat with the opposite arm and leg.

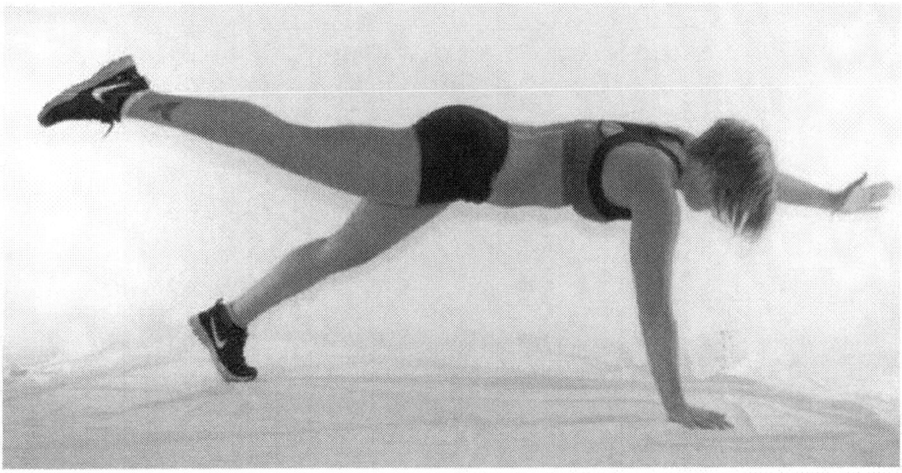

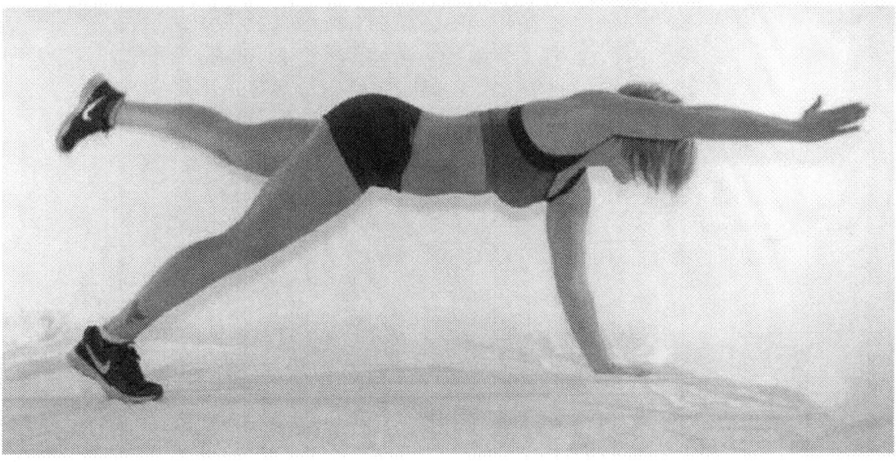

The Table Maker

This exercise will work your core while building strength and flexibility in your spine, back, triceps, shoulders, hips and buttocks. An advanced variation of this exercise that you might want to try involves not bending your knees and keeping your legs straight.

1. Begin by sitting on the floor with your back straight and your legs straight out in front of you. Place your palms beside your hips.
2. Inhale through your nose as you push your body forward until the soles of your feet are flat on the ground. Arch your hips and back and let your head fall backward.
3. Squeeze your back and abs tightly as you straighten your back as much as you can. Your goal is to make a table out of your body with your arms and legs at a 90-degree angle to your core.
4. Hold the table position for a beat and then lower yourself back to the starting position.
5. Repeat until fatigued. When you can perform between 10 and 20 repetitions of this exercise you are doing well.

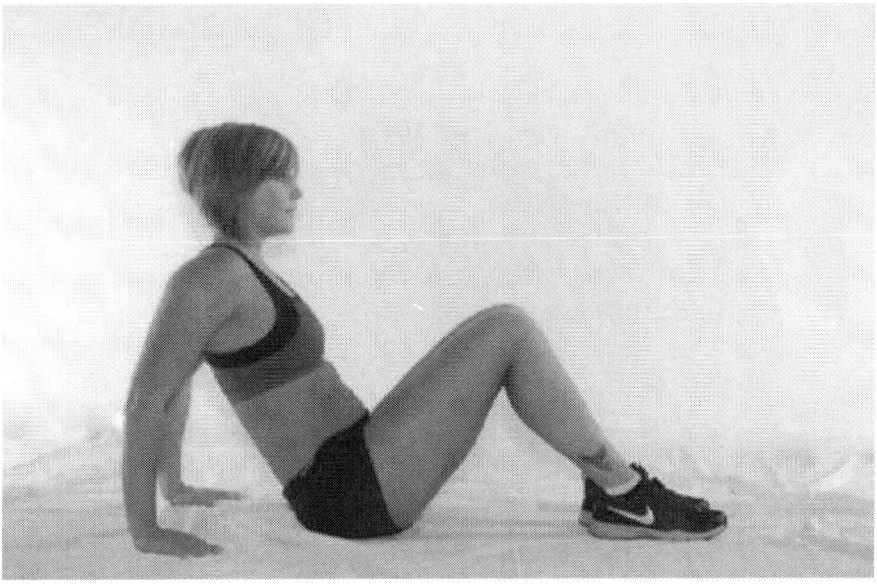

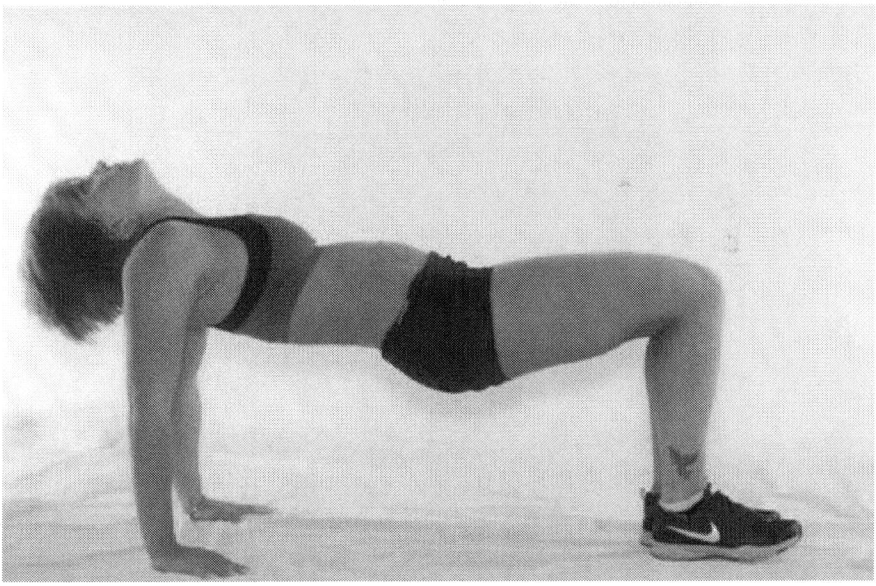

Back Bridge

There is no better exercise for strengthening and stretching the neck and back than the bridge. Sometimes called the wrestler's bridge, this exercise will also strengthen your abs, butt and legs while simultaneously improving your circulation, as well. I know how intimidating it looks at first glance but unless you have some kind of pre-existing medical condition, I urge you to give it a try. It really is one of the best bodyweight exercises out there.

Warm Up

In order to get your neck and spine ready to perform the back bridge, it is a good idea to warm up first by rocking back and forth. If you have never attempted to perform a full back bridge, you might want to stick with this warm-up until your neck strengthens and you get used to the motion.

1. Lie down on your back on a soft mat or carpet.
2. Position your feet close to your butt. Place your hands face down by your shoulders.
3. Press up with your legs so that you arch your back while driving your body backward.
4. Your weight should be supported by your feet, hands and the top of your forehead. Now rock back and forth so that you roll on your head. Your goal is to touch your

nose to the floor before rocking back to a more neutral position.

5. When you can rock back and forth ten times touching your nose to the mat, you are ready to move on to the back bridge.

Back Bridge

The only difference between the warm up and the full back bridge is that once you touch your nose to the mat, you will want to hold this position for a time. Your goal is to work up to holding this position for three minutes. Initially when you perform this exercise, your heels will likely come off the ground when you arch your back. As you gain flexibility, try to keep your feet flat on the ground. When you gain enough strength and confidence you can try performing the back bridge hands-free, so long as your nose is touching the mat. It is very important to never hold your breath during this exercise. Breathe freely and deeply at all times.

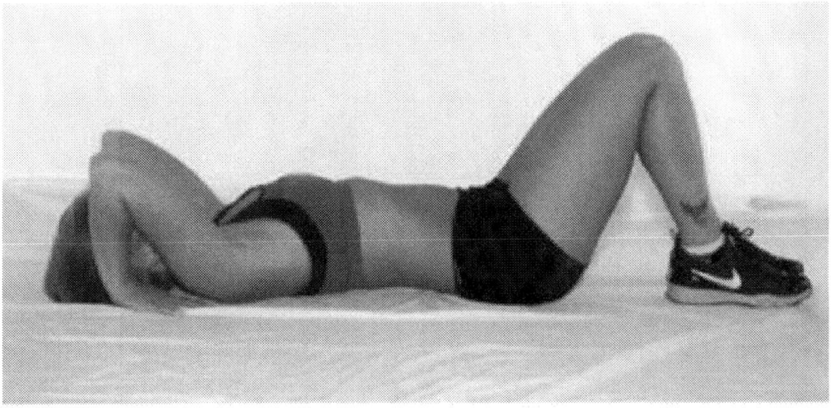

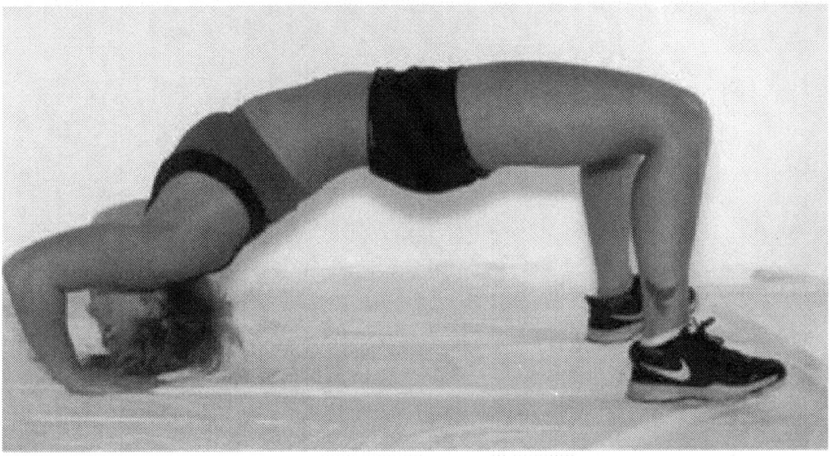

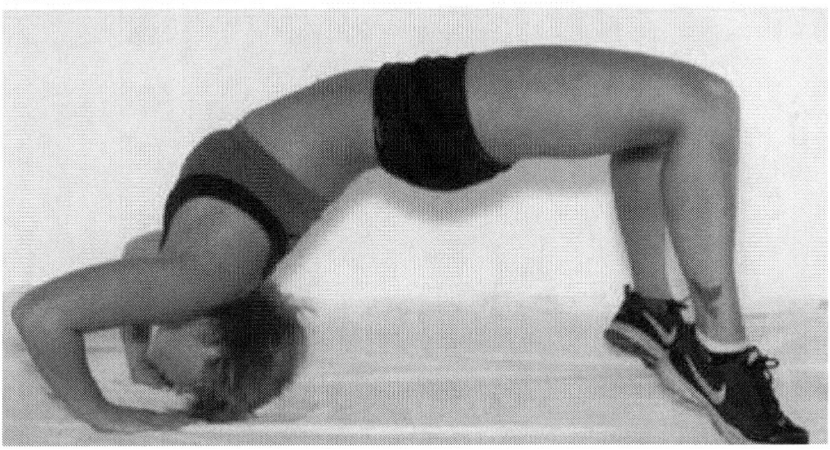

Gymnastic Bridge

The gymnastic bridge is a full body exercise that will build strength and flexibility in your shoulders, back, legs and abdominals. It is also a fantastic back bending exercise, which is why I've included it here. If you cannot get into the gymnastic bridge with your arms extended simply press up as far as you can go. With time and practice you will get stronger and you will still gain tremendous benefit by trying.

1. Begin by lying flat on your back with your legs bent and your palms by your shoulders.
2. Push off with your hands and legs, arching your back into the bridge.
3. Squeeze your butt and try to stretch your stomach as much as possible while using your legs to drive your chest forward.
4. Breathe slowly and deeply.
5. Try to hold this position for as long as you can. When you can hold it for a minute you are doing well. When you can hold it for 3 minutes you are doing fantastic.

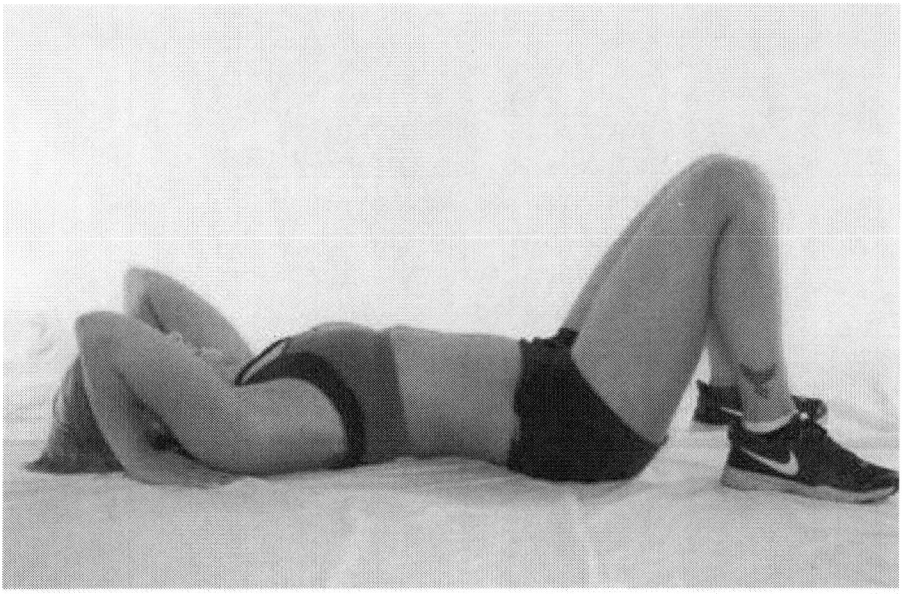

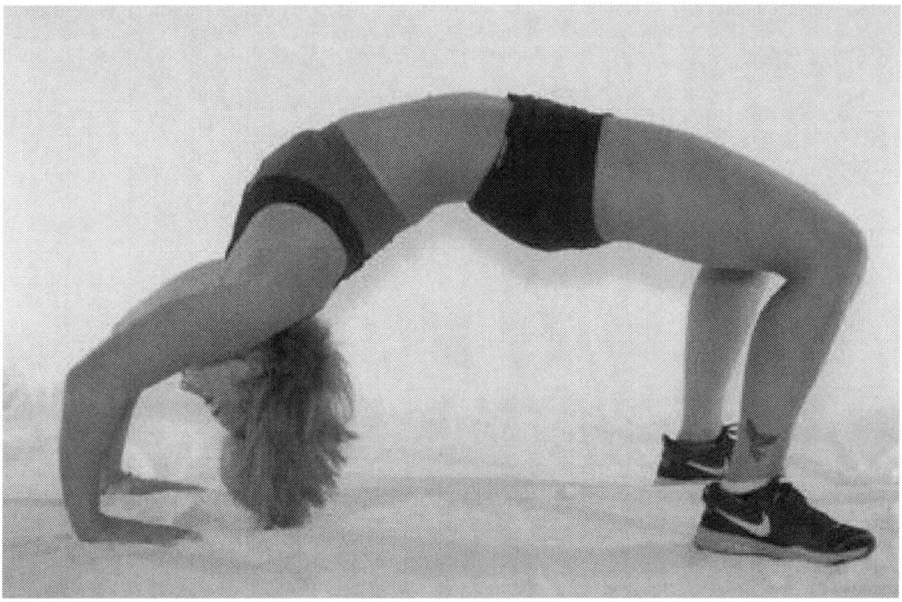

One Leg Gymnastic Bridge

Like its two-legged cousin, this core training exercise will sculpt and strengthen your entire body. The raised leg, however, will really force you to maintain your balance, which will really work your core muscles. You should only attempt this exercise once you have mastered the gymnastic bridge.

1. Begin by getting into a good gymnastic bridge with your arms extended and chest forward.
2. Lift your right leg up as far as you can. Try and keep it as straight as possible.
3. Squeeze your butt and tighten your abdominal muscles.
4. Hold this position for as long as you can while breathing deeply.
5. Switch legs and repeat.

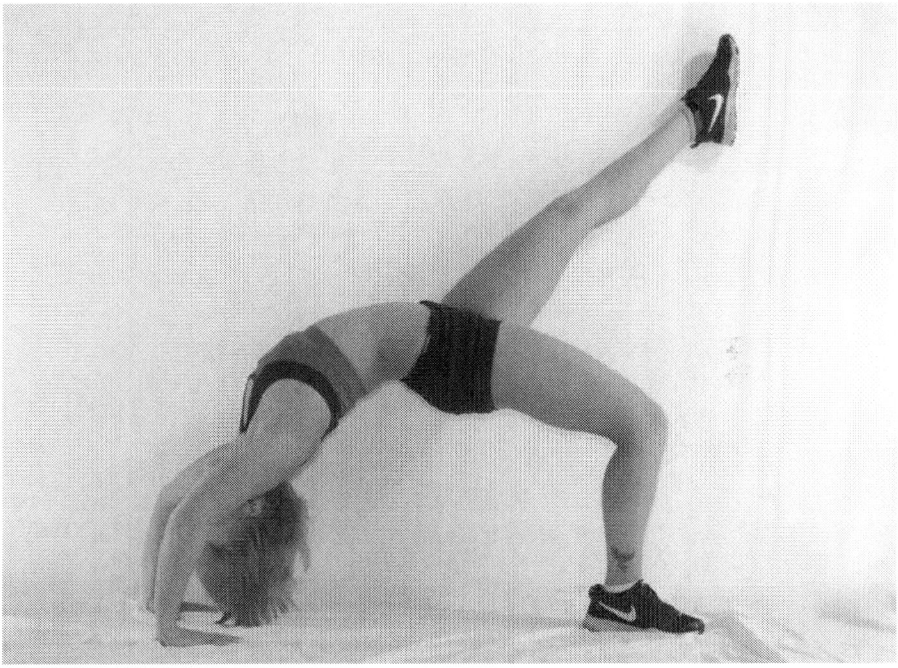

FAQ

Although I want real core strength I also want to look good and that means a six-pack. You mention how important diet is in achieving this. Do you have any further recommendations when it comes to diet?

Besides avoiding processed foods I think it is very important to avoid sugar. From my experience and research most people typically consume twice the amount of sugar that they should. When processed sugar hits the blood stream it will literally stop fat burning in its tracks. If you really want to follow a specific program I suggest looking at the slow carb diet that Timothy Ferriss developed. You can read about it on his blog here:

http://www.fourhourworkweek.com/blog/2007/04/06/how-to-lose-20-lbs-of-fat-in-30-days-without-doing-any-exercise/

Or you can check out his best-selling book The 4-Hour Body: An Uncommon Guide to Rapid Fat-Loss, Incredible Sex, and Becoming Superhuman which describes the program in much greater detail.

You can CLICK HERE to read more about this book

How much water should I drink?

Drinking water is important, but there is no need to become a water-drinking robot. There is a myth out there that most people should be drinking 8 glasses of water a day. This myth grew out of the misrepresentation of an US Air Force study done in the 50's which made the case that the average person needs 8 glasses of water a day. However, that water can come from a variety of sources, including other drinks like coffee or food. You don't need to drink a glass of water every couple of hours if you're not thirsty.

Having said that, it is important to remain hydrated. Water is obviously vitally important to the body, which is why we all possess such strong thirst mechanisms. What can happen though is that people who think they are hungry are actually thirsty, and they wind up eating high calorie food rather than drinking calorie free water. This makes sense, as most food is mostly water. For example, an apple is 85% water and a steak is 60% water. Your hunger pains may simply be your body trying to get water in whatever form it can. A solution for this is that if you are hungry, drink a glass of water and then wait an hour. If you are still hungry then eat something. I think you'll be surprised how often a glass of water can satiate your hunger.

How can I speed up the fat loss process?

You may want to look into my previous book The Bodyweight Exercises Bible. Some of the exercises in that book are excellent at burning fat, especially the squats and pushups. I would also recommend short, intense cardio sessions over slow, long distance cardio workouts like running. Hill sprints and skipping rope are excellent for this.

I have lower back pain and I'm having trouble doing some of the exercises. What should I do?

First of all make sure you see a physician before you start this or any other exercise program. You need to determine if you have any kind of pre-existing condition that might be causing you discomfort.

If the doctor clears you, start working on strengthening your core by doing the exercises in this book. From my experience the most effective exercises, when dealing with back pain, involve back bending of some kind. The issue that so many people have is that we are bending forward all day by typically sitting in a chair. The human spine is meant to move in all directions. Bending forward constantly causes tension to build, whereas, back bends can release that tension. Just make sure you go slow and steady at first with no quick or jerky movements. Be patient and gentle with your spine.

What do you think of diet sodas?

The problem with so many diet products is how people use them. They look at a can that says 0 calories and figure they can drink liters of the stuff. The truth is that although the can says 0 calories, there are still a lot of funky chemicals in there that can interfere with weight loss. From my experience having a glass or two at dinner is fine. If you are drinking more than that and are having difficulty losing weight I would suggest cutting way back on the diet sodas, if not eliminating them altogether. You are always better off drinking a glass of water anyway.

What program do you follow?

My basic philosophy is that I try and exercise everyday in some form. I don't follow any strict program, I simply do things. I do all of the exercises found in my books and I love doing hill sprints three times a week. I also like to do yoga.

What do you think of water fasts?

Water fasts typically involve only drinking water (no food or other kinds of drinks) for a 24-hour to 36-hour period. You can try this and it can definitely help with weight loss. However, I would recommend that if you feel physically ill at anytime, to break the fast immediately. Also, when you end the fast, don't do it with junk food. I suggest eating a salad and then waiting an hour before eating something more substantial.

What do you think of fruit fasts? I know a few people who lost a lot of weight this way.

I've tried 3-day fruit fasts before and they do work. However, I find them gimmicky. As well, by the third day, I typically felt lousy and the sight of fruit (surprise, surprise) made me sick. Some people swear by them but I don't recommend it. It's not a balanced approach.

What is the best way for me to figure out what works and what doesn't?

The best way is to keep a journal of some kind in which you'll record your workouts, what you eat and how you feel. We are all different. What works for one person may not work for you. By keeping track, you will see patterns develop and you'll be able to figure out how to do things better.

Further Reading

Convict Conditioning by Paul Wade

You Are Your Own Gym by Mark Lauren

Advanced Bodyweight Exercises by Patrick Barrett

Bodyweight Exercises for Extraordinary Strength by Brad Johnson

The 4–Hour Body by Tim Ferriss

About The Author

Anthony Anholt has been interested and involved in athletics and fitness for his entire life. His specialty is "gym less" workouts, or exercise systems that do not require any kind of special equipment. He is also interested in enhancing performance in all sports, but particularly basketball. This is his second book.

About The Models

Bry Jensen is a Vancouver based fitness model, personal trainer and author. Bry is available for fitness, glamour and commercial modeling work. She can be reached through her website at bryjensen.com or on Facebook at facebook.com/Bry.Jensen.Fitness

Jordan Rayburn is a Vancouver based fitness competitor and model. He can be reached through his Facebook page at facebook.com/jordan.rayburn

One Last Thing

You've now reached the end of the book and I hope you find it useful in building a better you. If you did find it useful I would very much appreciate it if you could take 5 minutes and write a short review for it on Amazon or wherever you purchased it. Even a couple of sentences would be immensely helpful to me. Regardless I want to thank-you once again for purchasing my book and I wish you all the best in the future.

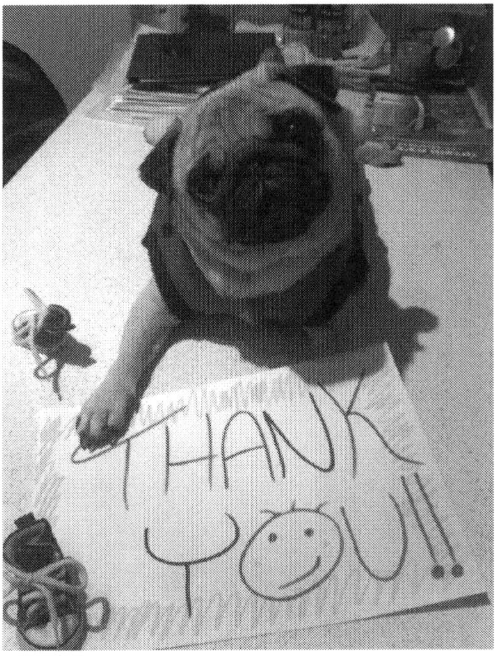

Printed in Great Britain
by Amazon

48655676R10077